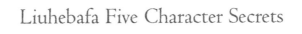

Liuhebafa Five Character Secrets

Liuhebafa Five Character Secrets

六合八法五字訣

※ CHINESE CLASSICS ※ TRANSLATIONS ※ COMMENTARY

PAUL DILLON

YMAA Publication Center
Wolfeboro, NH USA

YMAA Publication Center, Inc.
Main Office
 PO Box 480
 Wolfeboro, NH 03894
 1-800-669-8892 • www.ymaa.com • info@ymaa.com

20200215

Translation from Chinese by Zhuo Bing Yuan Pinyin
Romanization by Dr. Yang, Jwing-Ming
Cover Design: Katya Popova

Publisher's Cataloging in Publication

Dillon, Paul
 Liuhebafa five character secrets : Chinese classics, translations,
 commentary / Paul Dillon.—1st ed.—Boston, Mass. : YMAA
Publication Center, 2003
  p. cm.
  Presents the Five Character Secrets in its original Chinese.
Includes English translations and commentaries on the meaning of the
texts.
  Includes index.

  ISBN: 1-886969-72-8

  1. Martial arts—Psychological aspects. 2. Self-defense—
Psychological aspects. 3. Mind and body. I. Title.

GV1102.7.P75 D55 2003   2003109404
796.8/01/9-dc22   0309
                   QBI03-200241

Printed in USA

Contents

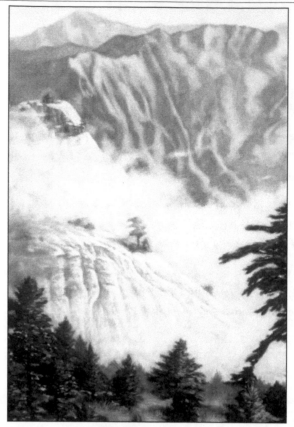

Hua Shan, 華山

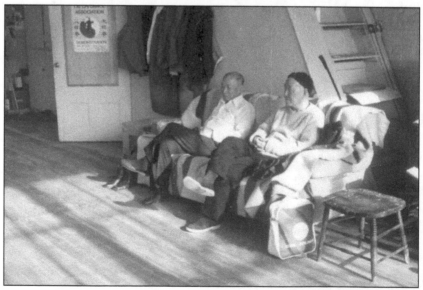

Mr. Li (left) and Mr. T. T. Liang (right)

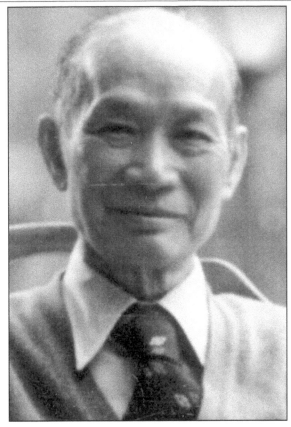

Li Zhong, 李忠

Huayue Xinyi Liuhebafaquan

The Five Character Secrets of Li Dongfeng are the original precepts of the rare internal martial art *Huayue Xinyi Liuhebafaquan*. *Huayue* means the remote mountain fastness of Mount Hua where the Daoist Sage Chen Tuan created the system. *Huayue* can also mean a beautiful place within that is difficult to find. *Xinyi* means Mind/Intent or the Creative Imagination (Higher Mind), a faculty of the True Self. *Liuhe* means the Six Combinations which describe the natural merging of body, mind, and spirit. *Bafa* means Eight Methods which describe how to experience the natural unification of the Six Combinations as a martial discipline. *Quan* means the art of boxing.

LINEAGE OF LIUHEBAFAQUAN

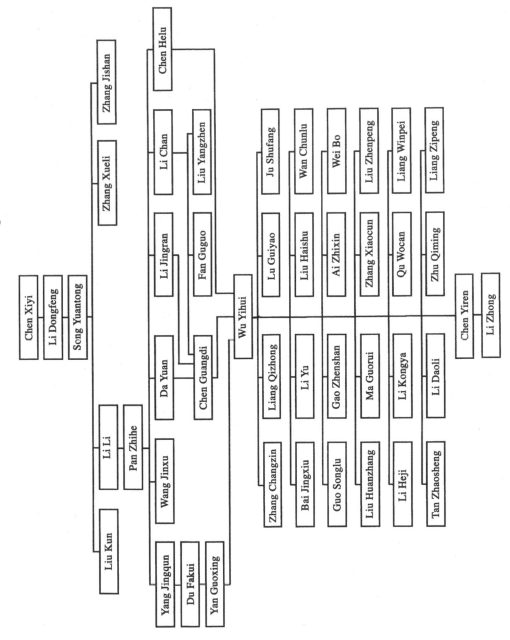

Chapter 1

From Chen Tuan to Li Zhong:

A Brief Overview of the History of Liuhebafa

The origins of Liuhebafa, also called Water Boxing, can be traced to the Daoist sage Chen Tuan (陳摶) (c.871-989 A.D.) also called Tunan and Fuyaozi. Chen is a mystical figure whose advice and perspective was sought by Chinese emperors during the period of the Five Dynasties and Ten Kingdoms (907-960 A.D.) and at the beginning of the Song Dynasty (960-1279 A.D.). In addition to Liuhebafa, he is credited with the creation of Taiji Ruler exercises, qigong and neigong systems that are still practiced today, and a form of Dream/Sleeping Daoist Yoga. Let's take a look at the life of this fascinating figure.

In c. 871 an unusual boy, often called a child prodigy, was born into a wealthy and high ranked family surnamed Chen. This child was called Tuan. His parent's estate located in Sichuan province was quite large and dotted by ponds and crossed by streams. Young Tuan was very much attracted to the water and could often be found walking or playing by the ponds or streams.

At the age of five, Tuan was playing by a pond one day when he noticed a beautiful bluish-green light moving toward him. Out of the light stepped the Immortal that Tuan called his Green Dressed Lady. The Lady took Tuan by the hand and said, "Look for me tonight in your dreams". She faded back into the light and then dissolved into the distance.

True to her words she came to him in his dreams that night and for many years to come. Through these visits the Lady took him to vast temples and places of learning where he began to study from the fountain of all knowledge. Of course he also had normal physical tutors who schooled Tuan in the Chinese classics such as the *Yi Jing* and *Dao De Jing*. This schooling provided an interesting counterpoint to the in-depth training he was getting by studying these works at a higher level. At these inner temples he could see and study the wisdom in its original form that had manifested as the *Yi Jing* and *Dao De Jing*. By seeing these works in their original form, he realized that his tutors merely repeated years of conjecture and commentary that had replaced any real understanding of these esoteric classics.

Following the expectations and wishes of his family, Tuan took the civil service examinations that would have placed him highly in the service of the emperor. He was already known as an authority on the classics; famous teachers in their own right came to confer with him. However, for whatever reason, he managed to fail the civil service exams. Not long after this apparent set back, both of his parents died. After an appropriate period of mourning, Tuan began to travel throughout Asia. This gave him the opportunity to study and confer with the great masters of the time.

Many years were spent at the feet of these teachers until he came to find hermitage in the Wutang mountains of central China. His retreat was called the Rock of Nine Rooms where the Five Dragon Immortals helped Tuan assimilate all that he had studied over the years. The time then came for the Immortals to test Chen Tuan. Each of the five in his turn, posed a question and as Tuan answered the last question successfully, he was immediately whisked away to his new retreat on Hua Shan, a sacred mountain in north-central China.

In a time when there was no mass communication it is surprising how quickly seekers after truth began to find Master Chen on Mount Hua. Amidst the cloud-shrouded peaks, Tuan endeavored to teach Chinese cosmology in its original simplicity. From his own direct experience, Master Chen taught that energy manifests as matter and that matter will return to energy. To illustrate this he outlined the process of birth, life, and death in the Six Combinations: Body combines with Mind, Mind combines with Intent, Intent combines with Energy, Energy combines with Spirit, Spirit combines with Movement, and Movement combines with Emptiness. The greater legacy of the Six Combinations is that it is a step-by-step method to move from the physical into a higher state of consciousness so that you can study from the same source as the old master himself.

During his hermitage on Mount Hua, the emperors of the time would often seek his guidance. But Chen Tuan would have none of it. He sought to live simply and explore the worlds of consciousness rather than the world of society. Nevertheless, the first Song emperor, Zhao Kuanying (r. 960-976, reigned as Taizu), appointed Tuan as an advisor to the court.

On the emperor's way to consolidate the northern regions of China, he stopped at Mount Hua to solicit Chen Tuan's advice with strategy in this campaign. Rather than compromise his ethics and serve in a campaign of conquest, Tuan offered a wager on a game of chess. If he lost, he would go with the emperor; if he won, the emperor would deed Mount Hua to him.

Tuan knew that the emperor was agitated by battle plans and distracted by affairs of state. This lack of concentration on the wager at hand cost the emperor the game and the mountain. Afterwards, Tuan revealed to the emperor that if his attention had not been in the past or the future, he might have won the game. He told the emperor that he was asleep and that he must awaken to the present. By focusing on the problem at hand, he would clearly see which step to take and that he must take one step at time. Following this advice, Zhao Kuanyin unified the northern kingdoms and ruled China in what would later be regarded as a cultural renaissance in China.

To this day, there is a monument to the contest between Chen Tuan and the emperor. It is located on top of the central peak of Mount Hua and called the Chess Game Pavilion. The second Song emperor, Zhao Guangyi (r. 976-997, reigned as Taizong), held Chen Tuan in such respect that he named him Xi Yi Xian Sheng meaning the unfathomable gentleman.

While on Mount Hua, Chen Tuan perfected methods to dream consciously. He would often go into a sleep state for up to one hundred days. From these forays into the dream world he discovered much and manifested it as practical methods for self-cultivation. From this repository of knowledge he created Liuhebafa and qigong methods that are still used today. For his many creations, derived from the dream state, he is still revered as the Sleeping Immortal.

One day, Chen Tuan called his closest disciple, Jia Desheng, and asked him to excavate a new cave in a nearby hillside. After some time, the cave was finished and Tuan moved in with all his belongings and manuscripts. It was in this cave that the master died. Some seven months after his death, his body was still warm and life-like and a multi-colored cloud stayed at the entrance. It was said that at night one could see a light shining from within the cave.

About three hundred years after Chen Tuan's death at the beginning of the Yuan Dynasty (1279-1368 A.D.), Li Dongfeng went off on a pilgrimage to Mount Hua (Hua Shan 華山). He was directed to some of the old caves and huts that Chen had used but there seemed to be a veil drawn over the exact location of Chen's last cave. Disheartened, Li resolved to give up the search and return home. That night, as he sat by his campfire, he noticed a light emanating from the side of one of the mountains. He anxiously made his way toward the light. His excitement was intense as he sensed the fulfillment of his quest. The light led him to the final resting place of the old mystic.

In that cave were all of Chen Tuan's belongings and manuscripts. Among those manuscripts were detailed instructions on Liuhebafa. Li who was a martial artist and a scholar proved himself to be a worthy student. Over the next months and years, with the help of the Daoist hermits there, Li mastered the intricacies of this internal art. Li then returned to Mount Yun (Yun Shan 雲山) to teach a small group of Daoists all that he had learned on Mount Hua.

Over the centuries, after Li returned to Mount Yun, Liuhebafa was taught only to a choice few. These fortunate students were usually chosen because they were adept in a martial art. These students brought their experience in styles such as Shaolin, Mantis, Xingyi, Bagua, and Taiji. The benefits of these arts were incorporated into Liuhebafa and made it a better and more complete art. In the Main Form, Liuhebafa already has the movements of Bagua; so a student with Bagua experience would simply enhance or emphasize that when performing the movements. Not unlike an accent, the inner person is not changed by the accent gained by moving to another locale.

During the Qing Dynasty (1644-1911 A.D.) people were aware of Taiji, Xingyi, and Bagua but Liuhebafa was almost regarded as myth. It took the Nationalist Revolution to bring some of the best martial arts masters to cities like Shanghai where Grandmaster Wu Yihui (吳翼翬) (1887-1961 A.D.) began to teach in the late 1920's. As Wu's fame as a peerless martial artist grew, so did the reputation of Liuhebafa as a preeminent martial art begin to grow.

In 1936 Wu took the position of Dean of Studies at the Nanjing Wushu College. After WWII, Wu returned to Shanghai and taught many students Liuhebafa.

Two of Wu's main students, Chen Yiren (陳亦人) (1909-1982 A.D.) and Liang Zipeng (梁子鵬) (1900-1974 A.D.), moved to Hong Kong at the end of the 1940's and taught Liuhebafa, Xingyi, Bagua, and Taiji. My teacher, Li Zhong (李忠) (1903-1982 A.D.) studied and explored Liuhebafa with Chen Yiren, Liang Zipeng, and others.

Li Zhong began his study of Chinese martial arts with the external systems. He was very adept at these arts and won the respect of martial artists throughout China. In his late twenties he was responsible for re-establishing the Jing Wu Martial Art Association (精武會) as a positive force in the martial arts community. He held the position of president of that organization for ten years.

As his reputation as a fierce competitor grew, he became known as the "King of the Hard Style". His last match in which an unfortunate incident occurred proved to be the turning point in his life. He left the external methods behind and put all of his attention on acquiring the internal method. He mastered the Wu and Yang styles of Taiji before moving to Hong Kong.

In Hong Kong he began his study of Liuhebafa under the tutelage of Chen Yiren. Chen left to teach in Singapore. So, Li Zhong began to explore the deeper aspects of Liuhebafa. This led him to several teachers that expanded his view and experience into Liuhebafa. He wanted to restore Liuhebafa to a more subtle and concealed art. Over the years, the external expression of the Main Form had taken on a Xingyi, Bagua, or Taiji flavor. Li Zhong enlisted the aid of Han Xingyuan (韓星垣) a Yiquan teacher who helped soften and round out the over-torqued and extended movements of Bagua and Xingyi that had crept into the Main Form.

In 1969 Li Zhong immigrated to the United States. He taught Liuhebafa in New York City, New Haven, Hartford, Providence, and his home base in Boston. Li Zhong taught that the core of the art, the principles, were of utmost importance. He maintained that Liuhebafa begins and ends in your dreams. *The Five Character Secrets of Li Dongfeng* was the foundation of all of his teaching and the inspiration for this work. Master Li Zhong passed away in 1982.

Chapter 2

Xingyi, Bagua, Taiji, and Liuhebafa

The approach to teaching and studying martial arts in China was based upon a monastic tradition that is characterized as door, hall, and chamber teaching. In times past the monastery, both Daoist and Buddhist, served as schools for medicine, the classics, and martial arts. The prospective student would come to the door of the temple and request to be taught the martial arts in that particular temple style. They might have to knock at the door many times before they would be allowed into a class that was taught outside the temple walls usually in proximity to the temple door.

If the student showed promise and had the proper demeanor, he would be taken into the training hall for further training beyond the instruction that he was receiving in the 'door class'. The hall curriculum expanded on physical conditioning and endurance. Usually the regimen included animal and weapons forms practice as well as much full-contact sparring to hone the fighting abilities of the student. At the higher aspects of the hall training, basic internal energy development training was begun. The ability shown throughout the training was of course weighed but it was the ability of the student to comprehend and succeed in the internal energy work that would be the deciding factor in the move to chamber teaching.

Chamber teaching was for the inner circle of students who would study directly under the master of the temple. It was to this group of advanced students that the master would impart the secrets of the system. This involved a more direct and user-friendly approach to the development of internal energy for fighting application and for the exploration of the esoteric dimensions of the art. The student soon discovered that this is where the true training began. All the other training, door and hall, was necessary and foundational but this is where the art was revealed both outwardly and inwardly.

About one hundred years ago this teaching model began to erode. As the Nationalist government replaced the Qing Dynasty, martial arts began to be available to the masses. The Ching Wu Martial Arts Association wanted to restore the culture and health of the Chinese people; but, as most things that are well-intentioned, the decision to provide a simplified form of Taiji proved to degrade Taiji and the other arts as well. Let's take a look at the three popular internal methods and how they relate to Liuhebafa.

Xingyi

Xingyi is an excellent bridge from external method to internal method. Of the internal methods Xingyi has the most to do with fighting. As with anything that appears simple it is very difficult to master. It is very quick, direct, aggressive, powerful, explosive, and forceful. The energy exhibited is linear and vertical that is developed from a strong rooting technique. The feeling I get from a Xingyi boxer is that of a freight train running full speed or an avalanche that sweeps away all in its path.

Originally Xingyi was very simple with only five forms or fists: Splitting, Smashing, Drilling, Pounding, and Crossing. The energy was compacted into the bones and muscles by focusing solely on each of the five fists as they were practiced over and over again. Over time other practices such as the Twelve Animals were added. There was also the attempt to overlay the practice with Daoist philosophy but this art has its origins in Buddhist thinking and Shaolin standing practices. This has led to some confusion regarding the basic underlying principles of the system. The key to Xingyi is to be spontaneous and let the subconscious (yi) respond with the appropriate form (xing). The spontaneity of Xingyi flowed out of the focused practice of the five fists. Auxiliary practice sets and philosophies tend to distract the mind into over thinking which slows the fighter. In combat, if you have to think about what to do, you've just lost.

Taiji

Taiji is the opposite of Xingyi in character. Where Xingyi is aggressive, Taiji is yielding and receptive. Taiji relies on circularity to neutralize and respond to an attack. The softness of Taiji is an illusion; it has often been called an iron bar wrapped in cotton.

This style also was originally very simple. It had only three forms. The intention was to develop the inner energy by keeping one's attention on a single point. By maintaining a single pointedness practicing the three forms tremendous power could be released on contact while appearing to have no power at all. This early training was then expanded into the thirteen forms that most Taiji enthusiasts are aware of. The forms were then increased to one hundred and fifty or more as well other training sets.

By the 1930's the art had been watered down by making it available to the masses. There were a few teachers who had trained in the old way and had great ability. They passed their Taiji on to a chosen few students; so, there is still real Taiji being taught, but it is rare. Unfortunately, Taiji, for the most part, has become a health practice.

Bagua

Bagua is still a premier fighting style. It can be hard or soft, aggressive or yielding. Bagua is movement, all kinds of movement. It can be linear and vertical or circular and horizontal. Blending with the movement of the opponent in harmony with situation and location. In other words, the Bagua practitioner blends with the total experience not just the attacker. This is one reason that it is a great system for dealing with multiple attackers.

Bagua is characterized by its practice of walking the circle. This simple exercise provides the foundation for the different combinations of forms or sets that later develop. The training methods of this style develop an incredible internal power.

As Bagua has spread throughout the world, we see some blending with Taiji, Xingyi, and other styles to detriment of the effectiveness of this art. There are, however, many orthodox teachers still teaching the methods that work.

Liuhebafa

Liuhebafa was the last of the internal methods to be taught outside China. Even inside China Liuhebafa had an almost mythic quality. Among the groups of inner circle students, Liuhebafa was graduate study in the internal arts. Within a style like Xingyi, for example, there were Inner Circle students. From within that group of students the best were chosen to study Liuhebafa; so it was an inner circle within an inner circle. This means, of course, that very few people studied Liuhebafa; but they were the best of the best. This insured that the art would remain intact because of the quality of student and the secrecy surrounding it. When you studied with one of these teachers, you were studying from someone of a very high level.

Liuhebafa is not so much different from the other three styles as the same. It has all of the power, aggressiveness, and directness of Xingyi. It has all of the yielding and neutralizing abilities of Taiji. It has all of the circling and enveloping power of Bagua.

At one time, all of the internal arts had similar training methods. Liuhebafa and Xingyi walked a circle before Bagua was created. Strength and endurance training was very similar; all of the arts used some kind of resistance training. Standing training was basic to all the internal arts.

Popularity is sometimes a curse. Taiji, Xingyi, and Bagua have become very popular and presented to many people. Sometimes, teachers would be 'certified' to teach who would not have the status of a 'door student' in older times. Sadly, much of Taiji and some of Xingyi and Bagua has been lost or watered down, as teaching these systems became a business or means of survival.

Liuhebafa is still rarely taught and for this reason it has retained its entire original training methods. Things like a moving or floating root that is basic to our training has been all but lost in the other internal methods. The main difference between Liuhebafa, Taiji, Xingyi, and Bagua is attitude and intent. In Liuhebafa you study, examine, and explore the Law of Cause and Effect (yin/yang) to reach a neutral platform or matrix so that you can objectively work toward establishing yourself in the Original Source and thus move beyond the worlds of matter. This is the point of the system as expressed in the Six Combinations (Liuhe). Our Eight Methods (Bafa) provide the tools to accomplish this.

From our perspective, Taiji, Xingyi, and Bagua seek to manipulate the energy through their understanding of the Law of Cause and Effect rather than truly blend with it. This approach keeps these practitioners cycling back through the same material experiences that the Buddhists describe as walking the Wheel of Awagawan. They tend to follow the first three combinations (body to mind, mind to intent, intent to *qi*) but are now reluctant to take or are unaware of the next step, which is to blend with Spirit. I believe that the other internal arts were originally oriented to combine with the Great Emptiness but lost much of this over time, as such training was not suitable for the students that were being attracted to these styles; Xingyi in particular attracted a rather coarse lot to be bodyguards and caravan escorts.

Liuhebafa uses external and internal training to strengthen and for-tify the body. It employs Chen Tuan's Dream Methods and contempla-tive exteriorization methods to experience those realms and dimensions that exist beyond the physical worlds. Liuhebafa is the next step for many in their training. As the student explores and experiences the methods of Liuhebafa, he understands that Liuhebafa has taken him through the threshold and that there will always be one more step to take.

Chapter 3
The Five Character Secrets of Li Dongfeng

Li Dongfeng (李東風), a scholar and martial artist, left his home on Mount Yun to seek Chen Tuan. While camping at the base of Mount Hua, Li noticed a light on the side of the mountain. When he went to investigate, he found the entrance to a cave. In the cave he found the illuminated remains of the old Sage along with detailed manuscripts that described Liuhebafaquan.

Realizing the importance of what he had found, Li decided to remain on Mount Hua until he mastered the material in the manuscripts. Some of the local Daoist monks helped Li Dongfeng to understand the principles and train in this new approach to the martial arts.

After mastering Liuhebafa, Li left Mount Hua and returned to his home on Mount Yun. He shared what he had learned with a small group of Daoists who lived nearby. After his return to Mount Yun, Li Dongfeng recorded all that he had learned on Mount Hua in one hundred and thirty-four verses (lines) of five Chinese characters per verse. His manuscript has become known as *The Five Character Secrets of Li Dongfeng* and is the only existing treatise today on the original principles of Liuhebafaquan.

The Chinese word for secrets in the title, *The Five Character Secrets of Li Dongfeng,* is *jue. Jue* carries the connotation of the oral tradition of passing the secrets of a system on to a chosen student. These special inner circle students were chosen only after many years of dedication and service to their teacher. They had proven to their teacher that they could be trusted to maintain the integrity and validity of their teaching.

Recording the physical, mental, and spiritual principles in a verse that could be easily memorized allowed the system to be passed on from generation to generation. This method of learning, however, is more than simple memorization. The verses being recited were taught and explained so that the student gained an understanding of that line. The verse then would become a seed that would bring forth the whole teaching when repeated.

In times past, the student was given one line at a time to study. The student committed the line to memory and then went about trying to understand its meaning. Although a line's meaning can seem obvious, there are many levels of understanding with each line. Since these lines are composed as contemplation seeds, they are meant to be dwelt upon.

In your study of these secrets, take one line and contemplate on it for a week. Keep a journal handy to jot down the observations and insights that you get as you go through the week. You will be amazed how the information will come to you. Set the tone of your study by picturing the master imparting the secret to you, his most trusted student. You might want to use the following story as a visualization exercise.

In a small neatly kept house, Master Li Dongfeng waited for his best student, Song Yuan Tong. Since Master Li had returned to his home on Mount Yun, he had been teaching Liuhebafa to a small group of Daoists. From this group Song had proved to be a worthy successor to Master Li.

Soon, a knock came at the door. "Come in, come in, and sit beside the fire, Yuan Tong." Not knowing why he had been summoned, Song hesitantly took a seat. "You have been with me for many years and I am very pleased with the way you have caught the true flavor of our art," Li said smiling warmly. "It is because of your integrity, understanding, and ability that I have called you here." Song was relieved that he had pleased his master but he was still puzzled. Li went on, "It is to you that I will pass the mantle of mastership. Tonight you will begin to learn the secrets of Liuhebafa, one verse at a time."

"Now, pull your chair over a little closer and repeat the line that I will recite." Excitedly, Song came closer to his teacher and Master Li began, "Mind/Intent is the basis of Methodlessness." Years later Master Song would repeat the same scene with his four top students: Liu Kun, Li Li, Zhang Xueli, and Zhang Ji Shan.

In the last line of *The Five Character Secrets*, Master Li Dongfeng reminds the student not to take these *Secrets* lightly. There is more here than meets the eye. It is wise to approach the *Secrets* with a beginner's mind. Imagine being beckoned to sit by the fire. Lean a little closer to better hear the master as he recites the lines that will open the doors of your mind and heart.

THE FIVE CHARACTER SECRETS
TRANSLATION GUIDE

心意本無法   ⇐ Chinese characters

XIN YI BEN WU FA

⇐ Pinyin romanization

Mind, Intent, root, without, method   ⇐ Word for word translation

Mind/Intent, root, no method   ⇐ Literal translation

Mind/Intent is the basis of "Methodlessness".   ⇐ Interpretive translation

Methodlessness is the state of doing without doing. In the state of Methodlessness there is no difference between what you are doing and that which is being done by Nature. When you are in this Total Harmony, you appear to be doing nothing, yet nothing is left undone. Your quest for this harmony begins with Mind/Intent.   ⇐ **Commentary**

15

1

心意本無法

Xin Yi Ben Wu Fa

Mind, Intent, root, without, method
Mind/Intent, root, no method

Mind/Intent is the basis of "Methodlessness".

Methodlessness is the state of doing without doing. In the state of Methodlessness there is no difference between what you are doing and that which is being done by Nature. When you are in this state of Total Harmony, you appear to be doing nothing, yet nothing is left undone. Your quest for this harmony begins with Mind/Intent.

In Liuhebafa, Mind/Intent is the Higher Mind, Wisdom Mind, or Creative Imagination. Higher Mind is a faculty of the Essential or True Self. Mind/Intent is the neutral point between cause (*yang*) and effect (*yin*). By attaining the neutral point, you can understand the ebb and flow of life so that you do not run contrary to it; you consciously cooperate with it.

Mind/Intent is not the physical will that originates in the reactive mind (subconscious and conscious). The physical will tries to force and manipulate; it is always reactive rather than active. The Higher Mind is active and creative and in harmony with the will of Nature.

To approach this study, leave your preconceptions behind. Begin with an open and child-like mind. As you progress in Liuhebafa, you find that this unique perspective allows you to go beyond technique; indeed, you become the technique.

2

有法是虛無

YOU FA SHI XU WU

to have, method, to be, empty, without
to have the method, to be, emptiness

Use the method of Emptiness.

Emptiness is clearing or emptying your mind of internal dialogue. For example, as you practice, remain focused on what you are doing and not be thinking about other things that need to be done. This clearing begins with thoughts that are obviously trivial. You then progress to more deeply rooted thought patterns that are a little more difficult to displace.

Your mind, like all of life, is constantly in motion. Don't use your energy to try to blank out your mind. You simply want it quiet enough to be able to hear the direction you're getting from your True Self through Mind/Intent. Just relax and be objective about your thoughts.

Don't treat Emptiness like a concept. Emptiness is a practice that you must exercise like any physical exercise. Try this exercise: Set a goal for yourself. Make a list of things you would like to see in your life, how you would like to change, or something you would like to accomplish; then pick one and totally focus on it. For example: You desire to explore Chen Tuan's Dream Methods and find out about the other half of your life; well, begin to place *all* of your attention on achieving this goal. Soon you'll find that study materials and methods will come your way, seemingly like a miracle. The thing to remember in this type of work is that you must be deliberate, methodical, and focused (single pointed). This type of thing takes discipline. Discipline means knowing what you want, truly want, and are willing to do what it takes to achieve it.

Remember that you are the causative factor in your life. What you envision will manifest. The objective here is to expand your conscious awareness so that you remember that you caused what is happening in your life so that you can be grateful for it; or if you don't like it, change it.

3

虛無得自然

XU WU DE ZI RAN

empty, without, to obtain, natural, certainly
emptiness, to obtain, natural state of being

Emptiness is used to acquire the Natural State.

It is natural for your body, mind, and spirit to be unified, combined, harmonized. When this total unity is realized it is called the Natural State.

To begin the unifying process that leads to the Natural State, use the following contemplative exercise called The Five Jewels of Liuhebafa. The five jewels are Relax, Empty, Calm, Still, and Natural. In the beginning, they appear separate but once mastered, you see that they are really one. Whether you are practicing moving or static postures, begin with *Relax* and let each jewel lead you naturally to the next.

Relax—let go of tension in your body from the top of your head to the soles of your feet.

Empty—quiet your mind of all internal dialogue.

Calm—with *Relax* and *Empty* you begin to feel an inner and outer tranquility.

Still—within this tranquility you find the Stillness in which the Inner Voice guides you.

Natural—by following the guidance from within, harmony comes into your life like water seeking its own level. The Natural State is not finite, you can never know all of it; therefore there is always another step to take.

Liuhebafa uses these five jewels at each stage of training, from beginning to advanced. From the beginning each movement begins with *Relax* and ends with *Natural*. In time, you will find that the beginning and ending are indistinguishable.

SUN, MOON, AND LIGHTNING EIGHT FORM STANDING

Standing practice is basic to the development of both internal and external skills in Liuhebafa. Some standing practices like the Twelve Pillars of Liuhebafa emphasize external strength development, unification of the whole body, and martial effectiveness. Other standing practices have more to do with the development of inner awareness of the relationship between the student's True Self and the underlying Life Force.

This practice is the latter variety. By tuning into the chakras or energy centers of the body, some people have immediate physical sensations such as immediate warmth and reddening of the hands and face. This is often accompanied by a tingling sensation. These sensations indicate the movement of the energy and blood out to the extremities following an expansion outward of one's consciousness. This is a benefit to your health.

One can often see light of different colors, i.e., pink, orange, blue, or golden. This light can flow in and out, blend together, or flash across your consciousness. You may also experience sounds such as the sound of distant thunder, the tinkling of bells, or the sound of bag pipes. Another sensation you might experience while standing is fragrances such as the smell of roses or various incenses. When you do experience these things, relax. Try not to focus your attention immediately on the thing that's happening. The more you can remain an observer the more intense the experience will become.

The title of this exercise is Sun, Moon, and Lightning Eight Form Standing and refers to the Sun, Moon, and Lightning Worlds that exist between the physical world and the next dimension (first level of heaven, astral world). In Liuhebafa, Chen Tuan's Dream Methods are usually the way the student first experiences this area of energy. This particular standing practice has also been very useful for students to link their dream experiences with their conscious waking state.

Follow the Five Jewels of Liuhebafa outlined in Secret number three to greatly enhance the benefits of this standing set. The following postures begin in the Wuqi stance. Stand naturally with your feet shoulder-width apart. Make sure that your knees are bent while doing the postures. Your shoulders should be down and naturally relaxed. Hold your head up with your chin slightly tucked in. Hold your tongue against your palate as if saying the letter 'L'. Hold your arms naturally by your sides. Breathe naturally throughout the exercise; never hold your breath. Stay in a posture for about one minute then gradually work up to five minutes or longer. You will be amazed at the results!

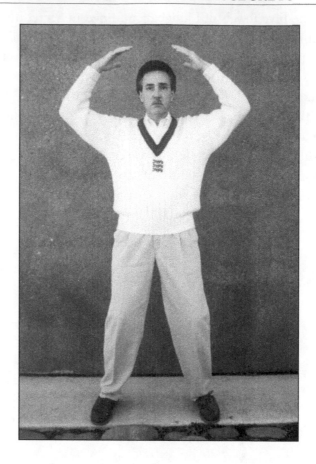

1. Crown Point (Top of your head)
From the relaxed Wuqi posture, raise your arms above your
head. Turn your palms toward you with your fingertips just
above your crown point. Your arms should be shaped like a
large circle.

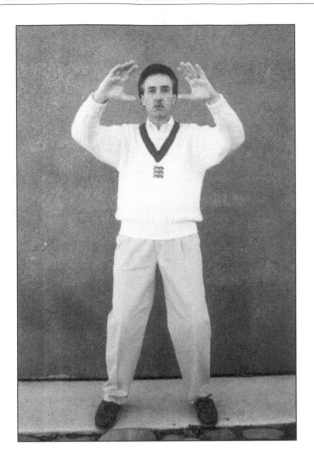

2. **Third Eye (Between your eyebrows; relates to the pineal gland in the center of your brain.**
   Slowly move your hands forward so that your palms press up and outward from your forehead. Keep the roundness in your arms.

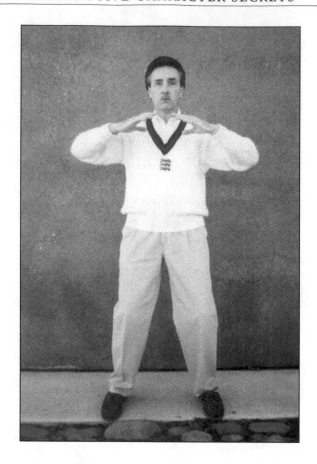

3. Throat (relates to the thymus and thyroid glands)

Turn your hands, palms down, and lower your arms to shoulder height. Be sure to keep the elbows down so that your arms form an arc.

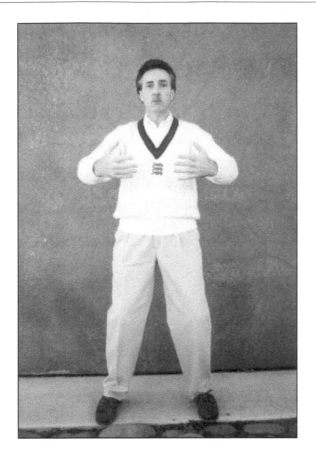

4. Heart

Turn your hands so that your palms face you and move your arms out as if you were holding a large ball against your chest. Hold your arms in a relaxed circle with your elbows slightly pointing down.

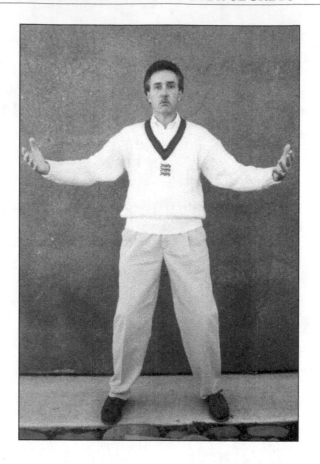

5. Scapula (Thoracic Hinge)

Move your arms outward as if the ball has been greatly inflated.

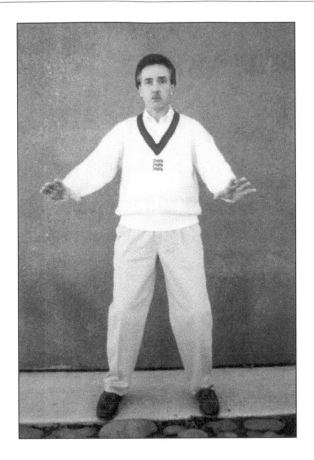

6. Spleen

Move your arms down and to the front of your body. Turn your hands over, palms down, and bend your elbows so that your hands and forearms are parallel with the ground. This posture is as if you are resting your arms on a counter or support.

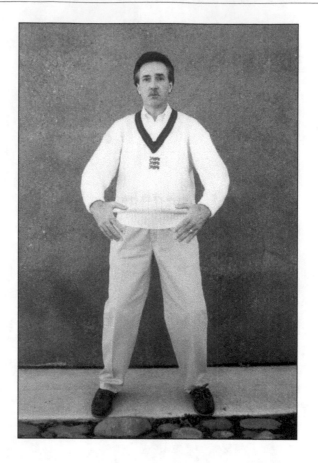

7. Abdomen/Dantien

Relax your arms outward from your waist into a large hold the ball posture, palms facing you.

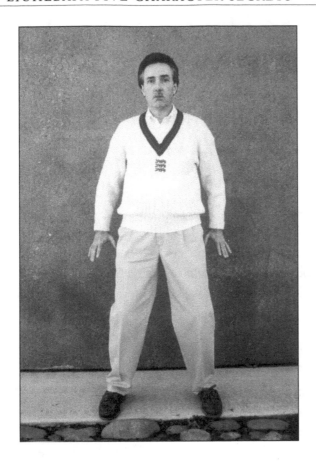

8. Base of Spine

Move your arms down and behind you, with palms facing the rear. You should feel as though you are pressing on a wall behind you.

While this is a standing practice, you can practice these postures while sitting. Make sure to use a straight-backed chair and keep both feet flat on the floor as you do the movements.

4

無法不容恕

WU FA BU RONG SHU

without, method, not, allow, forgive
without, method, not, to pardon

To be without a method is unforgivable.

If you were living in San Francisco and wanted to drive to Boston, you would be better served to have a map. Yes, you might be able to find your way to Boston if you drove east, but a map would make it a lot easier. Just so, the Natural State is not found by accident; you need a method.

The Six Combinations provide a map from the worlds of matter to the worlds of pure energy. The Combinations flow one into the other as naturally as streams flow into rivers and rivers into the sea. To follow this map, you must have patience. The understanding will not come all at once; it will come in stages or steps: Earth, Man, and Heaven.

The Earth stage represents your relationship to the external world. You learn that external physical functions are initiated internally. In the Man stage you learn that you have a creative relationship and responsibility with all Life. In the Heaven stage you learn that your destiny is to participate with the Life Force as a conscious co-worker.

THE SIX INTERNAL COMBINATIONS

1. Body combines with the Mind

The conscious mind (*Xin*) controls the movements and functions of the body. When in harmony, this relationship is intuitive and natural. As you relax to reduce tension, your physical body and your conscious mind will find a neutral point of balance between cause and effect so that your thoughts can clearly and succinctly be expressed through your physical actions.

2. Mind combines with Intent

The conscious (*Xin*) and sub-conscious (*Yi*) minds integrate to function as one unit (Mind/Intent, *Xin Yi*). By emptying yourself of internal dialogue, you open a pathway for reality to be shaped by your Creative Imagination (*Xin Yi*).

Your Creative Imagination, like energy, is invisible; nevertheless, this higher mind is the link between your True Self and your lower reactive mind. The Creative Imagination harmonizes with your other faculties to open the way to awareness or illumination.

3. Mind/Intent combines with *Qi*

When Body, Mind, and Mind/Intent come together, *Qi*, the force or energy that sustains all life is drawn to the activity to give it life and vitality. For example, if Mind were making vases, the vases would all be identical. The Creative Imagination uses the emotive quality of *Qi* to give color and distinction between the vases to make each one of them special.

4. *Qi* combines with Spirit

Spirit (*Shen*) needs *Qi* and *Qi* needs Spirit to be creative. So, when Body, Mind, Mind/Intent and *Qi* have come into alignment, then *Qi* naturally merges with Spirit to fulfill your Intent. You, the True Self, implant the seed (desire) into *Qi* that will manifest as form.

5. Spirit combines with Movement

Your expectation and desire become one. Everything in your outer world is created or actualized by inner movement. All of your thoughts, words, and deeds come from within the Stillness.

6. Movement combines with Emptiness

By following the Six Combinations, you arrive at the Original Source. You can now see, know, and understand in wisdom, power, and freedom. You realize that your destiny is to consciously work with the Will of Heaven. Expressing this harmony in your daily life is the Natural State.

THE SIX EXTERNAL COMBINATIONS

1. Neck, Spine, and Lower Back Combine.

Unification of your body begins with the spine. You have to be relaxed like a cat to be able to release instantaneous power. The secret is in straigthening and elongating your spine so that you can tilt the pelvis up; thus, tension can then flow down into your legs and feet thereby dissipating it into the earth. The action of this release of tension is called rooting. The effect is called *Song* in Chinese and means the dynamic state of relaxation.

By connecting the neck, spine and lower back, you promote the natural compacting of energy into your bones and bone marrow. With your body unified from the top of your head down to the soles of your feet (rooted stance), you are able to issue power or energy in all directions (*liuhe*).

2. Shoulder, Elbow, Wrist, and Hand Combine.

Your Heart/Mind and the joints are connected through the pericardium channel running from the little finger to your heart center. The posture of embrace produces a flow of energy that connects the brain with the sympathetic nervous system through the solar plexus or what we in Liuhebafa call the Citadel.

3. Hip, Knee, Ankle, and Foot Combine.

The Well of the Bubbling Springs energy meridian, located in the ball of the foot, is your connecting link between the Earth energy and your kidneys. The energy passing from the Well of Bubbling Springs to your kidneys passes through the bone marrow, which enlivens and rejuvenates the bones so that they can store the inner power, as power is stored in the curve of a bow.

4. The Three Smarts Combine (mind, eye, and hands).

Your mind is like the cat that quietly awaits his opportunity to pounce.

Await the chance.

Your eye is like the hunting eagle that seeks his victim.

Judge the chance.

Your hand is like a hungry tiger that snatches his prey.

Take the chance.

5. **The Nine Joints Combine (Wrist, Elbow, Shoulder, Hip, And Knee).**

When your Nine Joints are combined an energetic unity is accomplished. While the energy initiates your movements both in calm and conflict, the strength and power is concealed and is not obvious. You project an objective attitude that poses no threat to those around you. You simply appear natural.

6. **The Five Terminals Combine (Palms, Feet, Top of the Head).**

Applying the foundation methods of Liuhebafa unifies the Five Terminals with the Nine Joints so that everything will work together as one. Your joints are like step-up transformers through which the energy or force can flow from the solar plexus unimpeded to issue from the terminals. Again, this inner force is concealed not by some technique but by the attitude or demeanor that you have gained through your practice of Liuhebafa.

5

放之彌六合

FANG ZHI MI LIU HE

to let go, to arrive at, to fill, six, to combine
relax, to arrive at filling, everywhere

Relax in order to fill everywhere.

[Here LiuHe means the six points: north, south, east, west, zenith and nadir, i.e., all directions, everywhere.]

As you begin your practice relax your body from the top of your head to your neck, from your neck to your waist, from your waist to your knees, from your knees to your ankles, from your ankles to your feet. When your whole body sinks into the dynamically relaxed state, the

Vital Energy can fill every atom of your body. This is not a flaccid state; it is an active, alive, aware, and dynamic state. You can use the concept of a sphere residing in your solar plexus (heart center) that is radiating outward in ever expanding waves, sensing what is beyond the range of the normal senses and feeding that back to your sympathetic nervous system which then passes it to your brain for evaluation. In Liuhebafa we say that inside and outside are the same; so, as you advance in your ability to participate with the Life Force, your energy or spirit can fill the universe and beyond. Fill your universe within and without.

In this Secret there is also the sense of surrendering to the Life Force. Liuhebafa was originally known as Water Boxing to emphasize how you must flow and adapt as water does. Eventually, you will find that it is better to cooperate with the Life Force than it is to try to manipulate it. So, in this work, the best attitude to hold is that of water.

6

包羅小天地

BAO LUO XIAO TIAN DI

wrap, net, small, heaven, earth
to wrap up in a net, small, heaven and earth

Wrap up Heaven and Earth which are small.

As above (Heaven), so below (Earth). Have faith. What you hold in your heart manifests in your daily life. Today's thoughts and desires are tomorrow's conditions. So, choose carefully what you truly want in your life.

Through the practice of the disciplines and unified methods of Liuhebafa you can bring any goal into manifestation. Your goal may be lofty or mundane. The point is to exercise your innate abilities so that you can prove to yourself that you indeed are the motivating force in your life. There are no victims in Liuhebafa. This is a way to self-responsibility. The masters continually advise you to use your practice to make your world a paradise here on earth. Liuhebafa is a fantastically formidable martial art but you can practice it as a peacemaker, one who brings harmony. Yes, you can bring heaven and earth together and have peace in your own life. You must know, however, that this is a warring universe and as such there will never be an absolute peace established. This universe is ruled by the Law of Cause and Effect. The energy of peace will dissipate (die as all things do) and conflict will replace it. From the objective neutral point between cause and effect, you can use intention to make your life active and creative.

7

釋家為覺圓

SHI JIA WEI JUE YUAN

Buddhism, family, to be, to perceive, round
Buddhists, are perceptive, round

The Buddhists express their perception of the Natural State with a Circle.

This Secret lets you know that the practice and study of Liuhebafa can lead you home to the Original Source. You can move beyond the Wheel of Awagawan, the Wheel of Life, and find that there are worlds or dimensions that exist beyond the worlds of duality (*Yin/Yang*). And, most importantly, what your place or mission is in the scheme of things.

Lao Zi said that out of nothing came something and out of the something came all things. This nothing that he spoke of is the worlds of pure energy. The Buddhist travelers who explored these regions of the far country found that these areas are regions of pure energy and as such there were no comparatives to be able to describe their experience; so, they used the symbol of an empty circle to express their experience. They didn't mean that there's nothing inside, it's just that there are no words to describe it. Indians call this Anami, that which cannot be named.

In Liuhebafa you begin with the Dream Methods of Chen Tuan and advance to exteriorization methods in the contemplative standing practices. These are some of the methods that you can use to explore these inner regions for yourself.

8

道家說無遺

DAO JIA SHUO WU YI

The Way, family, to speak, without, to leave behind
Daoists, speak of, leave nothing behind

The Daoists speak of leaving nothing behind.

As you go into the Higher States of awareness, you understand that you must work in perfect harmony with the Life Force. The Daoists saw this as walking through this world in such harmony with the will of nature that they would leave no foot prints behind (leaving nothing behind).

The masters who walk among us go unrecognized. They are not hiding the fact that they are masters; but by their cooperation with the Life Force, what they do is only natural. They help and uplift those around them; but because they do it without fanfare or obvious activity, it is never noticed. An interesting exercise is to try to become aware of how your life has been affected positively in the past. Look at the cycles of your life. Start from the time you were born and consider what happened at that time with your family and in world events; then go by six-year increments to your present age. You will find the cusp of these cycles will contain the pivotal points in your life. Look for the underlying positive help that you got in those periods. The key to looking through your back pages is gratitude.

9

有象求無象

YOU XIANG QIU WU XIANG

to have, feature, to seek after, none, feature
have feature, to seek after, the featureless

Having Feature, seek afterward the Featureless.

You cannot help but be obvious as you first learn movements or exercises. However, once learned, seek your own harmony with the movement so that your movement will be totally natural and smooth.

Liuhebafa is a rich art, there is so much at the beginning that it can confuse one. Seek the calm and relaxed state when you begin so that you can move fluidly and let concern float away.

10

不期自然至

BU QI ZI RAN ZHI

no, a set date, natural, certainly, until
no set date, natural state of being, until

There is no set time limit in achieving the Natural State of being.

By holding in your Heart and Mind what you want and by constant, diligent practice, you *will* come into the Natural State. This is your birthright, to work hand in hand with the Life Force. You must understand that you are a unique individual and that your time frame is totally dependent on your experiences and what you have learned from them. You are on your own personal time track. No other person has the same time track, so there should be no need or desire to compete to get to a point before or at the same time as someone else. Simply relax into what you are practicing and learning and you will find your own personal way to the Original Source. What other goal is worthy of such effort?

11 & 12

要學心意功

YAO XUE XIN YI GONG

necessary, to learn, Mind/Intent, achievement
necessary, to learn achievement of Mind/Intent

先從八法起

XIAN CONG BA FA QI

first, to follow, eight, method, to begin
first follow, eight methods, to begin

If you want to learn the internal achievement of Mind/Intent, then you must first begin to follow the Eight Methods.

The Eight Methods are the result or the goal of Foundation training in Liuhebafa. Each Method is a quality of the Natural State. Through the Dream Methods of Chen Tuan, the Twelve Pillar Standing Postures in Three Levels, and Main Form training these Eight Methods refine into one consciousness as a whole rather than parts.

This internal achievement aligns you to your creative aspect so that you are directed by the True Self to Spirit, to Mind, and to Body.

THE EIGHT METHODS

1. Qi (Chi), Energy

These training practices show you that your thoughts move the energy, not vice versa. Through these participative methods, you understand that you initiate the movement of energy through you by your mind-set or attitudes; thus you arrive at a profound understanding of the Vital Energy and your relationship with it. You will then be able to harmonize your mind, movement, and breath to combine your *qi* with Spirit.

2. **Gu, Gu jing, Bone**

These methods teach you how to strengthen your muscles, ligaments, and tendons, and the overall structure of your body by enhancing the natural compacting of energy into your bones. Unifying your body through these methods facilitates and enhances your ability to issue energy.

These methods connect, align, and unify your skeletal structure of your body. This how you begin to unify body, mind, and spirit by first working with that which you can see and then working with that which is hidden.

You learn to coax the energy to penetrate your bones and marrow. This process is called marrow washing that cleans and renews the marrow. After your marrow is cleansed and the bones and joints are unified, your intent will be able to move the energy faster through your body. The more your health improves with this practice, and it will, the better able you will be to unify the energy that is both inside and outside your body.

3. **Xing, Feature or Shape, Assuming a Form**

You move from emulating a movement (usually of the teacher) to expressing the essence, or spirit, of that movement. Through this method you develop an attitude like water. An attitude like water can be described as coming into an understanding of yourself (by trying on other's shapes); thus, you become more aware of yourself and the creative/destructive power of attitudes and facsimiles.

4. **Sui, Follow, Blend and Stick to a Movement**

You learn to use both linear and circular methods of internal and external movement to intuitively blend with an aggressor. This training helps you overcome the fear of contact, so that your natural survival instincts can be harmonized to effortlessly neutralize, intercept, or evade an attack. Once you have brought your instincts into balance, then you can advance beyond instinctual response to the attainment of techniqueless technique. This level is termed the art of doing without doing by Daoists.

5. **Ti, Lift, Elevating the View**

Initially you will train to lift your head up as if suspended from above. This will stretch and elongate your spine so as to clear a pathway for the energy to flow unimpeded through your body. Again, step-by-step, as you achieve one level of unification, you move on to the next. And in the next phase of the training, you move your awareness up through your crown chakra to just above the top of your head. With practice you will gain a 360-degree viewpoint. This can be seen as a sphere of energy around the body that, among other things, acts as radar so that one can be immediately aware of imminent danger. After you gain a degree of ability with the 360-degree viewpoint, you will begin work on the techniques of exteriorization. Exteriorization means moving your awareness beyond the body in full consciousness. The training in this work begins with the dream travel methods passed down through our system from Chen Tuan.

6. **Huan, Return, Seeing Cycles**

With these methods you learn to work with the natural cyclic flows of energy inside and outside your body. In the beginning, you will have the feeling of gathering and releasing but it is the natural pulse of your body and you learn to cooperate with and utilize it. In time, through constant practice, you will realize that you want to be at the neutral point in these cycles. The neutral point is that creative point between yin and yang or cause and effect.

7. **Le, Restrain, Hold Back**

Your pathway to inner and outer harmony is found through emptying or quieting your mind. The quiet mind leads to the calm state. The calm state allows the Vital Energy to flow without hesitation. You will appear empty but you will be full. Conversely, you can appear full but will be empty, so that your opponent will fall into emptiness.

From the calm state, you have the advantage of being able to see when to seize the opportunity. You will be the expression of the law of sufficiency, using neither too much or too little power but exactly the right amount to achieve the purpose.

8. **Fu, Conceal**

Initially, your practice involves hiding or disguising your ability or intent until it is needed. However, as you learn to blend and harmonize with others, your abilities or intent will simply not be apparent. This 'skill' is more reliant on other's lack of awareness than on your attempt to conceal. Within these training methods is the secret of invisibility.

THE EIGHT EXTERNAL METHODS

1. **Qi Luo, Rising and Falling**

There are twelve breathing techniques or methods in Liuhebafa. All of our methods facilitate the movement of qi through your body, but the method you will finally arrive at is the Naturally Rising and Falling Breathing Method. By practicing the rising and falling method you will gain:
Song, a state of dynamic relaxation like a cat.
Your whole body will be fortified.
Spirit will be stored and concealed in your bones and joints.
Your energy will move from your Heart Center.
Your energy will flow unimpeded throughout your body.
Your strikes will be purposeful, crisp quick, and powerful.
You appear relaxed and calm, but you are always ready

2. **Dongjing, Moving and Stillness**

We say that inner and outer are the same, so you must learn to connect your inner awareness with your outer expression so that you can know when to act. This training is quite beyond the training of your instincts. You learn to move beyond your bodily animal instincts and operate from your Wisdom Mind so that you become aware of what your opponent is going to do the moment the first spark of his intention fires in his subconscious mind.

You see, this is not looking for an opening and attacking at once; that is the reactive approach. In Liuhebafa you learn to be the active imitator of the action. Through these methods you find that you find that your viewpoint comes from the top of the mountain.

3. Jin tui, Advancing and Withdrawing

Your decision to attack or withdraw is instantaneous. This method's emphasis is to have you work on maintaining your single-pointed focus on the situation at hand. In these situations you must maintain the heart and essence of a fierce tiger. Whether you are attacking or protecting, when you make contact your inner force issues at once; this gives your opponent no chance for escape.

4. Kaihe, Open and Close

You learn to gather and release your inner power or force through the practice of opening and closing. Initially, you release your power when you open and gather your power when you close. Eventually, however, you will be able to issue or gather power whether you are open or closed.

5. Yin/Yang, Inside and Outside

This method explores how the inside becomes the outside and how the soft becomes hard. You will see that each cycle arises as is needed and serves as balance to the cycle that went before and the one that follows. This training gives you insight into or sensitivity to opposing energies. With this perspective, you can blend opposites from one to the other to confound your opponent.

6. Xu shi, Empty and Full

This method teaches you how to conceal your stance or posture so that your intention is not made obvious by body language. When your hands are up they appear deceptively empty, but when you touch your enemy he knows your inner force is full.

7. Wa qiao, Jumping and Bridging

Your optimum contact distance is the length of your elbow to shoulder; we like to fight close because our techniques evolve into chin na or grappling. Use the method of jumping or bridging to close the gap and move inside or outside of your opponent. This method is simply about being in the right place at the right time.

8. **Liu he, Six Harmonies**

The three internal harmonies are:

Xin unifies with the Yi

Yi unifies with Qi

Qi unifies with Li

Where your mind goes the qi follows. If your Intent (Xin/Yi) is methodical, focused, and deliberate, your energy will flow unimpeded into all your movements.

The three outer harmonies are:

The shoulders unify with the Hips

The Elbows unify with the Knees

The Hands unify with the Feet.

Everything must work as one. This unity of inner and outer harmonies is called the Six Combinations. Also, this means the direction your energy travels, i.e., North, South, East, West, Nadir, and Zenith.

13

養我浩然氣

YANG WO HAO RAN QI

nourish, my, on a large scale, temperament
nourish, my, broad-minded, temperament

Cultivate the temperament of Righteousness.

This study gives you ever more freedom. With a greater freedom you must act with a greater sense of ethics and responsibility than ever before. Basically, you must not do anything that will harm others or yourself. To follow truth and live in harmony with all of life, it would be advisable to foster the Five Virtues in our life.

These Five Virtues are:

Discrimination—being able to choose what is good for you rather than what is not.

Forgiveness and Tolerance—the way to dispel anger.

Contentment—sufficient for the day is enough.

Detachment—by not being attached to things or desires, you are free to give and serve generously.

Humility—the balance to ego's negative aspects of arrogance and vanity

It is advisable at this point to also caution against the Five Passions; lust, anger, greed, attachment, and vanity.

14

遍身皆彈力

PIAN SHEN JIE TAN LI

entire, body, entirely, springy, strength
entire body, entirely, elastic and spring-like

The entire body is completely elastic and spring-like.

The foundation training methods of Liuhebafa employs the traditional methods of walking and rowing exercises using various postures. These exercises are a form of resistance training and are quite challenging. These methods require that you exert yourself, but the key to success is that you perform them in a dynamically relaxed manner. This is how your movements become supple and fluid. These methods allow the *qi* to settle into the marrow of your bones thus making our body elastic and spring-like from the inside out.

15

見首不見尾

Jian Shou Bu Jian Wei

to see, head, not, to see, tail
to see the head, not, to see the tail

The beginning is evident but not the ending.

You train to be featureless. Deception and inscrutability are the hallmarks of Liuhebafa. Your opponent thinks that he sees your power; but when he strikes, you are not there. He tries to grab you, but you are a ghost. You appear hard but you feel soft and vice versa. Our internal and external rooting methods have accelerated the compacting of energy into the bones so that you can appear relaxed and non-confrontative (what he sees at the beginning). When attacked, however, your energy issues immediately (what he doesn't expect) to the surprise and chagrin of your opponent.

16

無象亦無意

Wu Xiang Yi Wu Yi

no, feature, also, no, intent
featureless, also, intentless

Express neither Feature nor Intent.

You become an empty mirror for your opponent. Your goal is to not make your appearance or intention known. We begin this type of training by seeking inner and outer harmony by emptying or quieting the mind. The quiet mind leads to the calm state. From a calm state your energy that surrounds your body becomes subtle and less obvious. You will appear empty but you will be full. Conversely, you can appear full but will be empty, so that your opponent will fall into emptiness.

From the calm state you have the advantage of being able to see when to seize the opportunity. You will be the expression of the law of sufficiency, using neither too much or too little power but exactly the right amount to achieve the purpose.

Initially, your practice involves hiding or disguising your ability or intent until it is needed. However, as you learn to blend and harmonize with others, your abilities or intent will simply not be apparent. This 'skill' is more reliant on other's lack of awareness than on your attempt to conceal.

You know yourself but you do not want to be known. A study of Sun Zi's *Art of War* will further enhance your understanding of this Secret.

17

收放勿露形

SHOU FANG WU LOU XING

receive, to let go, not, show, form
receive, release, do not show form

Receive and Release without showing form.

By being non-resistant, you can receive or accept your opponent's energy to either let it pass through into the earth or return it to your opponent. Issuing or releasing your power takes much practice in receiving so that you can neutralize an attack. Neutralization, either by what you do or what your opponent does, is necessary for you to create an opening through which you may issue or strike with power.

Traditionally, Liuhebafa, like all of the original styles of Taiji, Xingyi, and Bagua, used joint hands or pushing hands exercises that trained you to interpret or feel the energy of the opponent. These exercises move from awkward to subtle so that you can receive and release without any preconceived idea of action to be taken (show form). Through this and further training you will find that your intention will be in the moment. Just so, your receiving and releasing shows no hint of form because it is instantaneous in that moment. What you do appears to be totally natural and in harmony with nature.

18

鬆緊要自主

SONG JIN YAO ZI ZHU

relax, tight, necessary, self, master
relax, tight, necessary, self-control

Your relaxing or tensing is necessarily self-controlled.

All of your movements are controlled by your will (intention). So, when you practice, use your will to relax and tense your movements. You can practice slow, fast, hard, soft or alternating between slow, fast, hard and soft. By practicing in this way you will be able to face all situations.

19

策應宜守默

CE YING YI SHOU MO

a plan, to respond, is necessary, to maintain, silent
a planned response, is necessary, to maintain silence

It is necessary to be Calm for a proper response to an attack.

Implied within this Secret is that you constantly reside in the inner silence so that you express the calm state. You will be as deceptive as the calm in the eye of a hurricane. From this neutral and objective point of view, you can see the situation with clarity and foresee any attack. Your calm state fosters your ability to act wisely in dealing with an opponent. If the danger is great, the more you will have to dig deep to be calm, but the more often you go to the calm place within, the more you will establish yourself there and move from responding to situations to living creatively in them. This calmness is featureless. In calmness, your ability is concealed.

20

不偏亦不倚

BU PIAN YI BU YI

no, inclining, also, no, leaning
do not incline, also, do not lean

Neither incline nor lean, remain straight in your stance.

In Liuhebafa you use your spine as a bow to issue energy or force. To do this, you align the top of your spine with the lower part of your spine. You take the arch out of the spine and straighten it so that you can let the body's tension relax downward into your feet and root into the earth. To straighten your spine, follow these alignments:

Bend your knees slightly.

Tilt your pelvis to pull the coccyx up and forward.

Raise your head as if suspended from above.

Keep your chin level; avoid tilting your head back or forward.

Keep your shoulders down and relaxed.

Let your elbows hang.

Keep your chest slightly concave.

21

視不能如能

SHI BU NENG RU NENG

look at, not, able, if, able
appear, unable, if, able

You appear unable, even when you are able.

Two high-ranking Karate black belts went to the school of a Taiji master to challenge him. The master who was across the room said, "You come closer. I am old. I cannot see. I cannot fight." Needless to say, when they got close enough for him to see, the only thing they saw was the wall and the floor.

It takes time to achieve this level of ability; but more than time, it takes you setting your intention (the image of what you want to be) at the beginning. You must have a picture and ideal of what you want to achieve and be.

One of the things that helped my imagination was Chinese martial arts movies. After training, I would go down around the block to the Chinese theater and catch a couple movies. They were all in Chinese with Chinese subtitles but I loved the action and the skill level. The ability of the martial artists in the movies inspired me to train even harder.

Study the methods of Feature, Restrain, and Conceal.

22

生疏莫臨敵

SHENG SHU MO LIN DI

raw, careless, not, near to, opponent
inexperienced, do not, get near to opponent

If inexperienced, do not engage the opponent.

If you don't practice regularly, you will gain nothing. Of course, this is true in any course of activity in life. So, don't be lazy. If you are lazy, don't engage an opponent; you will come to a bad conclusion. Anything worth doing is worth doing well. The more advanced a system the more practice you must put in to it. The magic comes from your enjoyment of solid, diligent practice. Rote practice of movement will lead nowhere, you must practice to gain knowingness and understanding. Then you will be able to face the opponent.

23

動時把得固

DONG SHI BA DE GU

to move, time, to hold, to attain, firm
when moving, hold, steadfast

Even during movement, use your energy to maintain a firm root.

It is important for you to build a strong foundation. In Liuhebafa you start in the legs to develop a strong root. Both Liuhebafa and Xingyi, arts from the same time period, build strength in the legs to develop a firm root. You use walking and rowing as the basic ways to develop this root. One of the unique things about Liuhebafa is that you can develop a moving or skating root, which means that even while moving you can issue the same power as if you were standing still. In the old days in China, students would train in rooting exclusively for three to five years before being taught anything else. That's how important rooting is.

24

一發未得人

YI FA WEI DE REN

one, to put forth, not, to attain, man
when issuing, do not, reach, man

When you issue energy (strike),
do not overextend yourself to your opponent.

This instruction carries on the idea of maintaining your center under all conditions. You must remain rooted outwardly and inwardly so that you maintain a balance of mind, body, and spirit. You do not want to extend bodily or you can be uprooted easily. Likewise, you do not want to overextend (broadcast) your intention, or your movements will be apparent and easily neutralized.

25

審機得其勢

SHEN JI DE QI SHI

judge, opportunity, to attain, near to, conditions
judge, opportunity, to reach, conditions

Look for the right time (opportunity) to make your move (attack).

Don't look for a confrontation. If faced with aggression, however, strike while the iron is hot. When you see your opportunity, you must strike at once, decisively. The longer you spar with your opponent the more opportunity you give your opponent. Remember that the first rule of combat is to not get hit.

If your opponent does not move, you are still. However, if your opponent moves, you will have already moved before him.

When you practice look to develop these three abilities.

1. The Eye. The ability to see your opportunity like an eagle looking for prey.
2. The Hand. The ability to grasp your opponent like a tiger.
3. The Mind. The ability to objectively watch for the opportunity like a cat watches a mouse

26

乘敵擊與顧

CHENG DI JI YU GU

take advantage of, opponent, strike, and, look after
take advantage of, opponent, strike, and look after [oneself]

Protect yourself and take advantage of the opponent by striking first.

Follow Sun Zi's instruction (*The Art of War*) to know yourself and know your opponent. Surprise is an advantage but don't be foolish. Review these instructions from above.

19. It is necessary to be Calm for a proper response to an attack.
20. Neither incline nor lean, remain straight in your stance.
21. You appear unable, even when you are able.
22. If inexperienced, do not engage the opponent.
23. Even during movement, use your energy to maintain a firm root.
24. When you issue energy (strike), do not overextend yourself to your opponent.
25. Look for the right time (opportunity) to make your move (attack).

This Secret also implies that you have become sensitive and aware through practice and can pick up the intent of your opponent. With such an awareness, you can have a preemptive strike that will end the situation quickly and cleanly.

27

剛在他力前

GANG ZAI TA LI QIAN

hardness, to be present, others, strength, in front
hardness is present, others strength, in front

In a confrontation, you may see hardness in the strength of others.

You will find that there are those experienced fighters who have trained in external methods and are very strong. These folks can be dangerous. Even more dangerous are those wily opponents who will show hardness to see what you will do or what you may know. If you are fortunate enough to realize that your strength is superior, end the conflict quickly.

Some internal artists may say that if your opponent is hard then you are soft or if your opponent is soft then you are hard. This position is a little simplistic especially when confronting an opponent of considerable skill. It is best to remain open and accepting so that you can receive their energy, hard or soft, and then in that moment respond appropriately.

28

柔乘他力後

ROU CHENG TA LI HOU

softness, take advantage of, others, strength, in back
softness, take advantage of, others' strength, afterward

Your softness will take advantage of your opponent's (hard) strength by leading it into emptiness.

In Liuhebafa you retrain and adapt certain instincts so that you don't oppose or resist and opponent. You do not run or withdraw; you are calm and waiting.

When someone confronts you, begin by listening to your opponent's energy. You can hear if their intention to do harm or not. Your calm exterior is misleading, making you appear vulnerable. When your opponent attacks, however, you can receive his energy, neutralize it, and redirect it. This leads your opponent into an off-balanced position in which he falls into emptiness.

29

彼忙我静待

BI MANG WO JING DAI

he, to hurry, my, quiet, to wait for
he is hurrying, I calmly wait

When he rushes to attack, I am quiet and calmly wait.

Standing practice is one of the ways to develop a rooted calmness. In time, you can see through an attack that is noisy and boisterous and look into the heart of your attacker. You can remain objective and calm and ready for any contingency. Diligent practice produces confidence and calmness.

It should be noted here, that in a confrontation time seems to slow down. You see things in a kind of slow motion. In a way it is as if you are watching someone else rather than participating in the experience yourself. To those observing the conflict, it might appear quick and over in the blink of an eye; but to you it took minutes to evolve. True training gives you a different perspective.

30

攻守任君鬥

GONG SHOU REN JUN DOU

to attack, to defend, to allow, a ruler, to fight
attack and defend, to allow, rule over a fight

You control the confrontation, you decide when to attack or defend.

Training in the inner and outer methods of Liuhebafa moves you past fear. Fear is rooted in ignorance and anger. The dream techniques and contemplative exteriorization exercises will bring an awareness of who and what you truly are. Thus ignorance is dispelled and anger is dissolved through understanding. You prove to yourself that you, the real you, goes on forever.

The first time I encountered a fearless person is when I met Li Zhong, Sifu. I pushed hands with him and was totally dissolved by his energy. Just facing a fearless person is disconcerting. You know that they are controlling the situation and will decide when it will come to a conclusion. Becoming fearless is the only option.

31

步步佔先機

Bu Bu Zhan Xian Ji

step, step, to take by force, first, opportunity
step by step, to overcome, at first opportunity

Methodically and quickly overcome your opponent.

When the balance or harmony of life has been disturbed by aggression or conflict, you have a responsibility to restore the balance. This is one of the dues you pay for understanding and participating in the Laws of Life through the internal methods of Liuhebafa.

So, when the responsibility for restoring harmony has been placed at your doorstep, methodically and immediately reestablish harmony. If this involves another person, then it is more kind to end the conflict quickly. Out of your centered calmness there can come a lightning bolt, one powerful strike and its over. Always use your training and experience with understanding and compassion.

32

時時要留意

SHI SHI YAO LIU YI

time, time, necessary, to entertain, intent
always, necessary, mindful

Keep your awareness (attention) on the business at hand.

In Liuhebafa we say that there is no past or future, only the present moment. This is the moment to place your attention in, the ever present now. So, whether you are training or fighting be deliberate, methodical, and focused here and now. You will find a great freedom in releasing that which you can no longer change and allow yourself to use your creative imagination to create the experience you want.

33

蓄勁如弓圓

XU JING RU GONG YUAN

to store, strength, like, bow, round
store strength, like, rounded bow

Just as strength is stored in the curve of a bow,
so do you store strength in the curves of your body.

Strength or force is concealed in the smooth curve of a bow. By walking, rowing, and standing you create the ability to release force from the curves of your hands, arms, shoulders, back, chest, legs, and feet. Continued practice not only emphasizes this storing ability but also conceals it from view.

34

發勁似箭直

FA JING SI JIAN ZHI

to put forth, strength, resembling, an arrow, direct and straight
issue strength. resembling an arrow, direct and straight

Issue your strength like an arrow, direct and straight.

Your movements, in relation to our opponent, may appear to be either diagonal, spiraling, or circling. However, your strength or force always issues out from your body in a straight line. Your body is unified through practice and, as such, acts in the most economical and efficient manner, which is in a straight line.

35

悟透陰陽理

WU TOU YIN YANG LI

to become aware of, thoroughly, Yin, Yang, principle
thoroughly become aware of, Yin/Yang, principle

You must thoroughly understand the Law of Opposites (*Yin/Yang*).

From the Original Source pure energy flows forth and splits into opposite forces, Positive (*Yang*) and Negative (*Yin*). From the activity between cause and effect, all matter and life is formed in this and other universes. This simply is the law of life.

You must go beyond simply observing cause and effect because this really is a circular process. Cause must become effect and effect must become cause. Birth, Life, and Death becomes Birth, Life, and Death the endless cycle of life that the Buddhists call the Wheel of Life or Wheel of Awagawan.

Work with and participate in the unseen force, Spirit. Spirit is the neutral point between *Yang* and *Yin*. This neutral point is the balance point, the fulcrum of creativity. This is the point where you take creative responsibility for your life in order to discover your True Self. It is at this point that you step off of the Wheel and onto the spiraling current that flows back to the Original Source, your True Home.

Cease to be reactive. Instead, live in creative harmony with life. Martially, no longer react to your opponent but move to maintain or restore harmony with him. Harmony is not so much a state to attain as one to maintain. There is always another step to take. Desire that your actions be as natural as the wind blowing through the leaves in a tree.

36

剛柔互參就

GANG ROU HU CAN JIU

hard, soft, mutually, to blend, to go close to
hard and soft, mutually blend, to go close to

Hard and Soft come together to mutually blend.

Out of hardness comes softness and out of softness comes hardness. Follow and use the precept of *Yin* and *Yang*, i.e., one begets the other. If your opponent attacks with hardness, neutralize that attack with circular softness. Move to a point where the strength of his hardness runs out, and then attack at that point of weakness. However, if your opponent attacks with softness (evasive circularity), attack with all force directly into their center like a tornado.

There are as many variations as there are people. Use your training to get to the Neutral Point between Cause and Effect, always respond actively never reactively.

37

調息坎離交

TIAO XI KAN JIAO

*to mix, breath, Water (the trigram of K'an), Fire (the trigram of
Li), to exchange
regulate breath, Water and Fire exchange*

**Coordinate your breath for the qualities
of Water and Fire to exchange.**

Through the breathing exercises of Liuhebafa Foundation, awaken
to your true nature. The use of the two trigrams (water and fire) suggests
that through the learning of life's lessons you can open the door to
awareness. Water represents Spirit and Fire represents the awakening
energy of awareness.

Physically, this refers to *Qi* (Fire, symbolic) in the *Ming Men*
(Kidney area) heating up the *Jing* (Water, symbolic) of the body to get
it to flow through the natural channels (meridians).

38

上下中和氣

SHANG XIA ZHONG HE QI

up, down, middle, harmonious, chi
up, down, middle, the chi is harmonious

No matter whether your breathing is up, down, or in the middle, the *qi* will be smooth and harmonious.

When you work hard, your breathing elevates. When you are at rest, your breathing is lowered. This is natural breathing. Through practice you train so that your breathing suits the activity but it is also calm and relaxed so that there is no impairment for the smooth flow of energy.

To get to this point requires hard work. Many folks in the internal method think that one can just move slowly and strive not to tax oneself. This is just not the way it is. Traditional martial arts use resistance methods and aerobic exercise. Carrying water from the base of a mountain to the top was more than an exercise in discipline; it fostered strength and endurance. The training methods of Liuhebafa are quite challenging and exhausting. Soreness has a new meaning. Li Zhong used to say, "First you ache then you shake, that's how the *qi* sinks to the bone". Hard work and dedication is the way to harmonious breathing.

39

守默為臥禪

SHOU MO WEI WO CHAN

to maintain, silent, to be, to lie down, Ch'an (Zen) Buddhist
to maintain silence, to be, reclining, Ch'an (Zen) Buddhist

Maintain the quietness and calmness of a Buddhist in repose.

To become aware of your True Self, you must be quiet and calm. In the stillness, you hear the Voice Within. Don't rush, there's no hurry. The secret to finding your Self resides in the relaxed state.

40

動似蟄龍起

DONG SI ZHI LONG QI

to move, resembling, hibernate, dragon, to rise
to move, resembling, hibernating dragon, to rise

Move like a dragon rising from hibernation.

When you awaken to your true nature, move slowly at first like the dragon awakening from its long sleep. Just as the dragon represents the power from heaven, you will find that you have the creative power to change your world.

The dragon is powerful and moves in an undulating and spiraling manner. Express your understanding of your power and creative energy in the Main Form. Emulate the beneficent and powerful dragon as it blesses the lives of those it touches.

The Methods of the Hibernating Dragon is another name for Chen Tuan's Dream Methods. By practicing these dream techniques, you become aware of the other half of your life. Thus you gain a higher, broader viewpoint and walk through life as one awakened, i.e., like a dragon rising from hibernation.

41

虛靈含有物

Xu Ling Han You Wu

empty, spirit, to embody, to have, substance
spirit of emptiness, to embody, to have substance

Within the spirit of emptiness is embodied the substantial.

Within the calm state your mind is free of all internal dialogue. You are free to focus or dwell upon your ideal within. This gives you an appearance of being insubstantial, but all the energy of the Life Force is embodied in this spirit of emptiness. Within you, hard and soft are the same; substantial and insubstantial are the same, and the beginning and ending are the same. Out of the neutral point between these apparent opposites flows a power that is unstoppable. This power flows like water into whatever you have placed your attention, the embodiment of the substantial.

42 & 43

窈窈冥冥趣

Yao Yao Min Min Qu

obscure, obscure, profound, profound, to hurry
very obscure, very profound, to hasten to

忽隱又忽現

Hu Yin You Hu Xian

suddenly, to conceal, also, suddenly, to appear
to suddenly conceal, also, to suddenly appear

As you hasten to become profoundly obscure (Spirit of Emptiness) you will be able to suddenly express or suddenly conceal (your internal force).

You are naturally evolving toward establishing yourself in the Natural State. Some folks will seem to progress slower or faster than others, but that is only natural. Water will seek its own level. The methods of Liuhebafa can help you hasten toward that state of being in which you seamlessly move through life doing what is to be done in the moment. In this state, you will be able to suddenly express or conceal the power within.

In Liuhebafa, you find the terms deception and conceal. What is meant is that those states are the natural result of the training. In other words, we don't train to become deceptive or hidden like some groups do.

You can't see the energy in a seed. When the seed is put into the proper environment, it germinates into a plant that does no longer resemble the seed. Follow nature's way and do not train to manipulate conditions in order to conceal or obfuscate a situation.

Look beyond the common concept of concealing. In North America, the Indians would learn to blend with the forest and animals so that they would seem to be invisible. You can learn to blend with the vibrations or consciousness of your opponent so that you will also seem to be invisible. You aren't invisible, but you aren't seen either. You can imagine the surprise of an opponent when an unexpected force explodes out of nothing.

This practice comes from the fourth Method; Follow.

44

息息任自然

XI XI REN ZI RAN

breath, breath, be responsible for, natural, certainly
breath for breath, be responsible for,
natural state of being

Regard every breath you take as being natural.

Train to gain stamina and naturalness in your breathing. Observe your breathing during strenuous activity; your breathing and heart rate are elevated. This is natural. Being natural is doing what is necessary in the moment. When you realize this, then you can accommodate going from one activity to another, i.e. activity to rest.

45

避免敵重力

BI MIAN DI ZHONG LI

to evade, to avoid, opponent, heavy, strength
evade and avoid, opponent, heavy strength

Evade and avoid the heavy strength (attack) of an opponent.

Training mitigates your ego. It is wise when faced with a formidable opponent who is apparently stronger or has the advantage to take the path of least resistance. Don't meet hard with hard. Soften your response to interpret and receive his energy. Yield and move to a position of strength. It takes tremendous energy to mount a heavy attack. Let the opponent dissipate his energy and power. The training of Liuhebafa teaches you how to yield to, evade, redirect, or absorb heavy strength leading it into emptiness.

46

原來自我始

YUAN LAI ZI WO SHI

an origin, to come, self, me, to start
origin comes, the subjective ego, starts

You are responsible for every action.

Whether you do well or not in a confrontation is totally your responsibility. To be able to do what you want to do, you must embody the precepts of this system through diligent practice.

Remember, what you do today will become tomorrow's conditions.

So, when aggression becomes conflict, what you do in the moment will dictate what the next moment will be.

47

雙單可分明

SHUANG DAN KE FEN MING

double, single, can, distinguish, clear
double and single, can, distinguish clearly

Make the difference between double and single [weightedness] clear.

Simply put, single weightedness is when your body is in total balance. You can be either static or in motion, either on one leg or two it doesn't matter because you've found the harmony. This harmony is taught in the Foundation methods of Liuhebafa. Through these methods you make sure that all of your postures are internally connected so that no matter which way you move you are in balance, single weighted.

Double weightedness is either not achieving or the falling out of balance.

48

陰陽見虛實

YIN YANG JIAN XU SHI

Yin, Yang, to appear, empty, solid
Yin and Yang, to appear, empty and solid

Yin and Yang manifest in both the empty and solid.

Yin and *Yang* are always present together. *Yang* needs *Yin* to manifest and *Yin* needs *Yang* to manifest. One cannot exist without the other.

So, they are always present in all that is manifested. So, you can be both hard and soft, empty and solid, or inner and outer at the same time.

Yang is depicted as a solid line, and *Yin* is depicted as a broken line. By combining these solid and broken lines into three line combinations, you will come up with the eight trigrams or *bagua*. These eight trigrams are then combined into sixty-four hexagrams and are the foundation for the *Yi Jing*. The relationships that are expressed through the trigrams and hexagrams will give you the insight into the many manifestations of cause and effect and how to deal with them from a purely objective viewpoint.

49

虛引敵落空

Xu Yin Di Luo Kong

empty, to lead, opponent, to fall, empty space
empty, to lead the opponent, to fall into empty space

Emptiness can be used to lead an opponent to fall into a void.

The more you discard, the more empty you become. This is called investing in loss. When your opponent attacks, you sink into your center to evade, redirect, intercept, or neutralize. You only give your opponent what you want him to have.

Initially you learn to physically move and blend with your opponent. Later at the advanced stages you blend with his consciousness so that you seem to disappear. He attacks air. You simply aren't there. The stronger the attacking force the deeper into the void the opponent will fall.

It should be noted that it takes a lot of energy to blend with the consciousness of an opponent. It is much easier to blend into the surroundings like a building, trees, or a crowd. The old hermits went off to live in caves or by lakes and oceans. They found it was less difficult to deal with a solitary lifestyle. Your challenge is to be able to live and evolve in society. By learning to blend with life, society, and our environment, you can contribute positively to the world consciousness.

50

欲收放更急

YU SHOU FANG GENG JI

to desire, to receive, to let go, to change, hurried
to desire, to receive or release, quickly change

It is desirous to quickly change
between Receiving Energy and Releasing Energy.

Don't play with your opponent. Blend with your opponent to interpret his energy and then receive (accept) his energy in order to redirect, absorb, or neutralize it. When the point of neutralization (off-balancing) has been reached, release your energy quick and as straight as an arrow.

Learning to stick and discharge is important in single combat but absolutely necessary when facing multiple attackers. Move into position to deliver one devastating blow or technique to end the conflict. Drop them when and where we hit them.

51

兩腿似弓彎

LIANG TUI SI GONG WAN

both, legs, to resemble, a bow, curved
both legs, to resemble, a curved bow

Both legs should resemble the curve of a bow.

Over and over again in foundation, it is stressed that your legs should curve, that is, always be bent. The curve is seen from the side. Consciously keeping your knees slightly bent builds the leg strength to support the pelvic tilt so that your spine can straighten.

You store power in your legs. By straightening your spine, you can issue that power fully and effortlessly. Remember, store strength like a rounded bow. Make sure that your knees are bent and flexible this will allow you to root so that your strength will flow from the soles of your feet to your solar plexus.

52

伸縮腰著力

SHEN SUO YAO ZHUO LI

to stretch out, to contract, the waist, to exert, strength
stretch and contract, the waist, to exert strength

Stretch (Open) and Contract (Close) the waist to exert strength.

In Liuhebafa we when we speak of the waist, we are mean the solar plexus. This area that is the upper part of the waist (diaphragm) is also seen as the Heart (*Xin*) Center through which we become conscious of the world around us with our emotional senses. By placing your attention on the solar plexus, called the Citadel, and consciously stretch and contract the diaphragm, you enhance your ability to effectively issue force through any part of the body. Much time needs to have been spent opening and closing the area around the diaphragm while in standing practice to nurture the ability to issue force.

53

脊臂須環抱

Ji Bi Xu Huan Bao

the spine, the arm, must, to encircle, to embrace
the spine and the arms, must, encircle and embrace

Your back and arms are rounded into a circular embrace.

This instruction aptly describes the Embrace the Tree standing posture. By rounding the back and arms you also make the chest slightly concave. This posture stimulates the *Ming Men* or Gate of Life at the base of the Thoracic Hinge as well as the pericardium channel that runs from your little finger through your palm to the Heart Center. By opening the arms into an expansively round embrace and then closing them into a more definite circle in front of the body, you are able to pump the energy to the fingertips. Feeling this movement of energy through your body prepares the way for issuing energy skills to be developed.

54

內外混元氣

Nei Wai Hun Yuan Qi

internal, external, to mix, original, chi
internal and external, to mix, the Original Chi

Mixing the Original Chi is always from within (internal to external).

Following the previous instruction, by moving into postures that pump the energy through the natural channels of the body you find that the energy flows from the *dantien* (abdomen) to the other points of the body. Foundation practices open and cleanse these natural pathways for the energy to flow. When the body is in tune, energy flows automatically from the *dantien* and could be considered an autonomic function.

When you consciously move upward from the abdominal area and begin to work from the Heart Center, the Third Eye, and Crown Chakra you then become a transformer of energy rather than a storage battery.

Dantien in today's martial art circles usually refers to the energy center that is two to three inches below your navel and back near the spine. This center is responsible for the body's energy and sustenance. In Liuhebafa, dantien encompasses and unifies three areas: the lower *dantien* (abdomen) related to Earth, the middle *dantien* (heart) related to Man, and upper *dantien* (head—third eye—crown chakra) related to heaven. Earth, Man, and Heaven are interrelated and inseparable. Just so, the three areas in your body are interrelated and inseparable; from the top of your head to the soles of your feet, there is one unified elixir field.

55 & 56

息念要集神

Xi Nian Yao Ji Shen

to put a stop to, to remember, necessary, to gather together, spirit
to put a stop to remembrances, necessary, to gather the spirit together

彷佛臨大敵

Fang Fo Lin Da Di

resembling, like, near to, great, opponent
similar to, being near to, a great opponent

A way to halt wandering thoughts so that you can focus is to act as if you are facing a great and famous fighter.

There is much that is continually going on within you. Some of your thoughts are profound and some are trivial. When you practice or face an opponent you must focus and marshal all of your activities toward a goal. This is not unlike a symphonic orchestra that has many talented artists but need a conductor to lead them in one concerted effort.

It is well to keep in mind an old saying, "When you practice, see yourself successfully facing a great opponent. And when you are fighting an opponent, act as if you are practicing".

57

目光如電流

MU GUANG RU DIAN LIU

the eyes, bright, like, lightning, to flow
bright eyes, flow like lightning

Bright and full of life, your eyes move like lightning.

Your initial training works to increase your peripheral vision making it more acute. The next stage trains your intuitive nature and increases your range of vision past physical boundaries.

The awareness that comes with this enhanced vision is evident in your eyes. They become full of life. On the positive side, such eyes can reassure and comfort one. On the dark side, such eyes can fill one with dread and foreboding. Your eyes are windows of the Soul. What do you wish others to see in them?

58

精神顧四隅

JING SHEN GU SI YU

subtle, spirit, to look after, four, corners
spirit, looks after, the four corners

Your Higher Awareness encompasses 360 degrees.

Your Higher Awareness is always awake, reaching out, sensing in all directions at once. Through the techniques and exercise methods of Liuhebafa, you can quiet your reactive mind and begin to tune into your Higher Awareness. When you were a child, you could hear and tune into your Higher Awareness; but as time and socialization happened, you turned your attention more to the mundane and trivial things of life. In time, by residing in the stillness, you can turn your attention back toward the light and sound. This is a process of discovery and exploration. The training methods of Liuhebafa can give you the tools to dig for the rich treasures within.

59

前四後佔六

QIAN SI HOU ZHAN LIU

front, four, to the rear, to seize, six
front four, to the rear, seize six

Keep 40% in the front leg and 60% in the rear leg.

Strength is stored in your legs. In China, students in Liuhebafa would row (leg exercise) for at least three to five years to develop a strong root in their legs and feet before they would train in other movement. The 60/40 weighting shows the strong emphasis on the back leg strength in this style. In time, however, the weighting will be interchangeable because unity, balance, and single weightedness are the result of dedicated training.

60

掌握三與七

ZHANG WO SAN YU QI

the palms, to hold fast, three, and seven
the palms, control, three and seven

Your hand strength lies 30% forward and 70% back toward the body.

Reserve 70% of our strength to protect your body and use only 30% to attack. You are tapped into the vast energy reserve of the Life Force. So 30% is more than a substantial amount of force needed to neutralize an opponent.

This style is likened to a dragon whose power comes from heaven. The dragon's body is powerful. It uses its legs to contact the foe, grasps with its claws, and then uses its twisting body to overcome the foe; but the power issued comes from the heaven (Life Force) within.

61

形動如浴水

XING DONG RU YU SHUI

form, to move, like, to bathe, water
the form moves, like, bathing in water

When you do the Form, move like you are swimming in water.

As water flows into every space, so should you move fluidly and continuously with a calm intent. Once you have mastered the choreography of the movements, then the contemplative nature of the exercise becomes apparent. In a real sense, the movements bathe the mind, cleansing it of useless and trivial thoughts. It is from this objective state that you can comprehend the point of your own creativity.

62 & 63

若履雲霧霽

RUO LU YUN WU JI

to be like, actions, clouds, mist, the sky clearing up
to be like, the actions of cloudy mists, the sky clearing up

飄飄呼欲仙

PIAO PIAO HU YU XIAN

floating, floating, to greet, to desire, Immortal
airy and graceful, to greet, to desire to be like an Immortal

Move like clouds and mists clearing in the sky,
As you float gracefully to greet an Immortal in the clouds.

The ultimate goal in Liuhebafa is to discover the way of return to the Source, your True Home. Immortals are folks just like you and me who have found the Way and are willing to help you find the way home. There are many Immortals that the Chinese revere, but in Liuhebafa you can look to the Five Dragon Immortals who taught and tested Chen Tuan and Li Dongfeng. They are known by a color, which is their title: Green Dragon, Red Dragon, Orange Dragon, Blue Dragon, and Golden Dragon.

You can visit the Temple of the Five Dragons in the contemplative state. The Secret gives you a clue as to the modus operandi. Find a comfortable place to sit or recline. Take some time to breathe and relax. Empty your mind of extraneous thought. Feel a calmness coming over you as you settle into the tranquility of your inner stillness. Close your eyes and gently look at a point between your eyebrows.

Place your attention on going to the Temple of the Five Dragons. The temple is set into the side of a low hill with its roof rising above the ridge. The countryside is green, verdant (the color is more vivid than you can believe). There are beautiful low, sculptured-looking pine trees that line the road leading to the temple.

The temple is of classic Chinese design with the peaked pagoda roofs. The temple has five levels. Each level is painted with the specific color that is associated with each of the Immortals. The first level is green followed upward respectively with red, orange, blue, and gold.

At the entry to each of the levels there is an instrument which, when sounded, will summon that Immortal. So, walk up to the entry of the green pagoda. Beside the first doorway is a small instrument that appears to be drum. Strike the drum with your hand. The sound you hear is that of distant thunder and carries your attention to the center of the room just beyond the portal.

The room is much larger on the inside than it is on the outside. In the center of circular room is a shaft of glowing emerald light.

As you gaze at the light, the Green Dragon Immortal steps out from the glow. Without words he asks you what you are seeking. Search within and then ask him how to find your heart's desire, and just listen.

You begin your training with these Immortals under the tutelage of the Green Dragon. When you are ready, you will be passed to the next Immortal for their particular gifts. So, move like clouds and mists clearing in the sky, as you float gracefully to greet an Immortal in the clouds.

64

浩浩乎清虛

HAO HAO HU QING XU

great, great, in, pure, empty
very great, in, pure emptiness

You will find the Majestic Greatness in pure Emptiness.

The more you discard the more you gain. As you discard images from your conscious reactive mind, you open the way for your True Self to assume control of your life and actions. This principle is often called emptying the cup.

65

意動似懼虎

YI DONG SI JU HU

idea, to move, resembling, to fear, tiger
the idea of the movement, resembling, a fearsome tiger

Your Creative Imagination (Intent) moves like a fearsome tiger.

A tiger on a hunt is single pointed, totally focused on its prey. When it moves it is awesome in its ferocity and power often bringing down animals that are larger and more powerful like a water buffalo or an elephant.

Just so, you must use this example of focused intensity when you are establishing your intention or goal. You must have the strength of purpose to stick to achieve this goal. Do not think that something is too big

LIUHEBAFA FIVE CHARACTER SECRETS

or too difficult to accomplish. Through experience you will see how holding onto your dream and steadily working at it can bring the most fantastic results.

66

氣動如處子

QI DONG RU CHU ZI

qi, to move, like, a young lady
qi moves, like that of a young lady

Your *qi* moves calmly like a gentle young lady.

The more you practice the methods of Liuhebafa the more calm and graceful you become. The expression of *qi* in your movement will be more fluid and flowing. This, of course, changes you and your life. Your friends will notice that you are easier to be around because this unique exercise has begun to remove your rough edges. You start as a cube with the destiny of becoming a smooth ball.

67

犯者敵即仆

FAN ZHE DI JI PU

to invade, he who, opponent, immediately,
to fall prostrate
he who invades, opponent, immediately
fall prostrate

As soon as the opponent moves to attack, he will immediately be knocked down.

Your training will prepare you for all contingencies. You will learn to wait calmly, but with certainty. If your opponent does not move, you are still and calmly wait. If your opponent moves, you will have already resolved the conflict.

68

五總九節力

WU ZONG JIU JIE LI

five, chief, nine, joints, power
five chiefs, nine joints, power

The power flows through the five terminals and nine joints.

The foundation exercises of Liuhebafa unify your five terminals and nine joints so that they will work together as one. Your joints are like step up transformers through which the energy or force can flow to issue from the terminals.

The Five Terminals
Two Palms, Two Feet, Top of the Head
The Nine Joints
Two Wrists, Two Elbows, Two Shoulders, One Pelvis, Two Knees

69

欲學持有恆

YU XUE CHI YOU HENG

to desire, to learn, to grasp, to have, persevering
to desire to learn and grasp, to have perseverance

If you want to learn and understand, you must have perseverance.

Perseverance to us means more than sticking to something and seeing it through. In other words, you don't want to just tough it out. If this is something you really want to do, then you must have a plan. First sit down and think about what you really want to see happen with yourself and this art, what *you* want to get out of it. Now, write this down; and if you have several things, prioritize them. Set up a plan for your classes and practice sessions. Give yourself at least one day off a week. You must keep a journal of your practice, classes, contemplative exercises, and diet; this is a must! Most of all, you must enjoy this. You have to be having fun or you're not doing it right. If you are having a problem, go back and review your journal. You'll see where you need to put the effort or slack off a bit. Remember, its all about harmony and balance.

70

升堂可入室

SHENG TANG KE RU SHI

to advance, hall, can, to enter, room
to advance into the hall, can enter the room

You must advance into the hall before you can enter the (Master's) chamber.

Follow the methods of Liuhebafa step by step, first things first. Keep in mind that you must practice systematically. Don't try to rush ahead in your training. Follow the plan that your teacher lays out for you.

In ancient China students would begin their studies outside the temple near the door. The monks would come out and teach a very basic martial art. The students who did well and showed promise were brought inside the temple to learn in the main practice hall.

Those few students who did well in the practice hall were then brought to study directly with the Master of the temple. When you came into the Master's Chamber, you would learn the secrets of the system that were reserved for a precious few to carry on the system.

Liuhebafa is called the Last of the Closed-Door (Master's Chamber) Systems because it was kept so secret and hidden. It was a closed-door system within closed-door systems.

71

顯隱無與有

XIAN YIN WU YU YOU

to display, to conceal, without, and, to have
to display and conceal, having and not having

Your appearance of having or not having inner force will be displayed or concealed naturally.

There is energy or power constantly around you, but you can, through ignorance, be impervious to this reality. You could not continue in your life without this Life Force to sustain and nurture you. Indeed, but for the Life Force there would be no life to live. It usually takes a catastrophe like a tornado, hurricane, or earthquake to notice the power that is all around you.

The more advanced you become in Liuhebafa the more you become aware of your inheritance, to be one with the Life Force. You don't become it; you are already it. You just have to realize it. When you do, then you become unnoticed by most people until you display that energy. This is why the masters work in the silence. They aren't silent; it's just that the people around them aren't sensitive enough to recognize their activity.

72

疑神尋真諦

YI SHEN XUN ZHEN DI

to doubt, spirit, to seek, true, to investigate
a doubting spirit, to seek, to investigate the truth

Have a spirit of skepticism as you seek to investigate the truth.

The study of Liuhebafa requires that you research the roots of the system. Investigate and study both the internal and external aspects of this art.

Don't take anything for granted. Don't just blindly accept what a teacher tells you. Take everything with a grain of salt until you can prove it for yourself. The methods of Liuhebafa give you the tools to discover the truth for yourself through direct experience. The light of truth shines brightest in those who began the quest for truth with a skeptical mind.

73

妙法有和合

MIAO FA YOU HE HE

wonderful, method, to have, harmonious,
to combine wonderful method, to have, harmonious combinations

This wonderful method (Liuhebafa) combines all movement harmoniously.

The Liuhebafa Main Form is a long practice set. Over time the masters have refined and improved this practice set so that your movements can be more fluid and harmonious. All movement is interrelated; like a dragon, one part cannot move without all parts moving together. This means that body, mind, energy, and spirit all moving together in unity. When you move one part, everything moves. When you are still, everything is still. This produces efficient, effective, and economical movement. Eventually, you and the movement are one.

74

離神空虛寂

LI SHEN KONG XU JI

to separate, spirit, space, empty, solitary
to separate the spirit, empty space, solitary

Separate the spirit with emptiness and solitude.

When you use your Creative Imagination to pursue truth or set a goal, this is called separation. By emptying your mind of reactive and useless thoughts, you come to points of separation. At these points of separation you discover your True Self and your relationship to Life. The first major separation is discovering the 'mysterious pass'. The 'mysterious pass' is the neutral point between *yin* and *yang* where you understand that the spirit of creativity is within you.

Separation happens in the stillness, solitude. Solitude is that quiet place within where your consciousness is anchored even amidst the sometimes-chaotic pulse of life.

75 & 76

拳拳得服膺

Quan Quan De Fu Ying

to clasp, to clasp, to attain, to wear, the breast
hold closely, to attain, to wear on the breast

道理極細微

Dao Li Ji Xi Wei

the way, principle, extremely, fine, subtle
the principle is the way, is extremely fine and subtle

The way to these principles is extremely fine and subtle. It is wise to keep the secrets you attain to yourself.

My teacher didn't mind letting people watch our classes. He would say that they could see but could not understand. So it is with fine and subtle truths. Keep the energy of these truths within to propel you toward new and deeper awarenesses; don't dissipate your energy by sharing your hard-won insights or truths with those who do not or cannot understand. Don't cast your pearls before swine.

77

欲動似非動

YU DONG SI FEI DONG

to desire, to move, to resemble, without, to move
to desire to move, to resemble, without moving

When you are moving, desire to appear as though you are not moving.

There is a saying that smooth waters run deep. There is much hidden power stored in moving slowly, calmly, and effortlessly. This follows the instruction, "When you move, move like a river. And when you stand, stand like a mountain". This is a high level but attainable with practice.

78

靜中還有意

JING ZHONG HUAN YOU YI

quiet, center, still, to have, idea
center of quiet, still have the Idea

Within the center of your stillness, maintain your Intent.

You live in a world where people live darkly, blind to reality. They have lost all knowledge of who and what they truly are and spend their time on unworthy goals. Instead of looking for the light, they bury themselves in the darkness of forgetfulness.

It is not easy to pursue the high path in such conditions. As you walk among the people of the earth, keep and foster your intention at the still-point within. When you are able to quiet outside thoughts and distractions, you will find the Great Stillness. Within the Great Stillness, you will be able to maintain an objective viewpoint under all conditions.

79

息念氣自平

XI NIAN QI ZI PING

to put a stop to, to remember, chi, self, even
to put a stop to remembrances, your chi, even

Cease wandering thoughts and the flow of your *qi*
will become calm and even.

Watch your wandering thoughts and just simply observe them as if you were sitting on a porch watching the traffic go by. Don't stop the thought; watch it go by. This process will remove energy from these passing thoughts and they will eventually go away.

If you get involved with your wandering thoughts, you waste your energy and send it in all directions thus losing all focus. Keep your energy in your center.

80

默默守太虛

Mo Mo Shou Tai Xu

silent, silent, to maintain, great, empty
silently, to maintain, Great Emptiness

Silently maintain the Great Emptiness.

There is an old Daoist saying, "The contemplative's heart is like a calm lake undisturbed by the winds of society". When you find the Great Emptiness, you realize that it is not empty but complete and full. There is great joy in knowing what the words 'to be' mean.

81

元根築基法

Yuan Gen Zhu Ji Fa

the first, a base, to build, a foundation, method
the first basic to build, a foundation, method

The first step in learning this system is building a firm foundation.

The Foundation methods of *Wai Gong*, *Qi Gong*, and *Nei Gong* are absolutely necessary in training your body, mind, energy, and spirit. *Wai Gong* nurtures the strength and vitality of your physical body. *Qi Gong* nurtures the inflow and outflow of energy through your body. *Nei Gong* nurtures the dialogue between your physical self and your True Self. Trying to go immediately to form work without taking the time to practice the Foundation methods is like building a house on sand.

82

蘊藏皆珠玉

YUN CANG JIE ZHU YU

to collect, to conceal, all, pearls, jade
collect and conceal, all, pearls and jade

Collect your pearls and jade, but keep them all concealed.

It is best to remain silent about the great truths that you learn. It is by your living the truths you have discovered that they are shared with others. Example is always the best teacher.

83

說難亦非難

SHUO NAN YI FEI NAN

to say, difficult, also, is not, difficult
said to be difficult, also, is not difficult

Liuhebafa is said to be both difficult and not difficult.

When everything around you is telling you that the truths within this system do not exist, it takes great effort to remain objective and to keep your eyes on the prize. As you see these truths manifest in your practice and your life, the road becomes easier. This system proves itself to you by direct experience.

84

看易本非易

Kan Yi Ben Fei Yi

to look, easy, root, without, easy
to look easy, at origin, not easy

Things usually aren't as easy as they first appear.

It will take time, dedication, and faith to achieve the benefits of this method. It can be done but problems do arise at a certain points in your practice. It is at these points where you have to give up lifelong patterns and habits. Rather than confront bad habits directly, place your attention squarely on the training methods and exercises. This will remove the energy that supports the habits and behavior that are giving you a problem. Then you can reaffirm the goal you wish to achieve and the methods that will get you there. You can succeed if you put all of your heart and mind into it. Remember, the only difference between a rut and a grave is the depth.

85

有志事竟成

YOU ZHI SHI JING CHENG

to have, determination, an endeavor,
to finish, to succeed
to have determination, an endeavor,
to finish and succeed

In any endeavor, you must have the determination to finish and succeed.

Any endeavor should be something you *want* to do; however, when you do take on a task have the discipline and self responsibility to give it your absolute best effort.

There can be no progress until you make up your mind to practice. You must always keep forging ahead into new material. The new material keeps things fresh and helps you to understand what you have previously learned.

86

世間無難事

SHI JIAN WU NAN SHI

the world, in, without, difficult, an endeavor
in this world, without, difficult endeavor

In this world, there is no endeavor that is difficult.

You create your own world. When you impress your desire into Spirit, you must know that it already exists and will manifest physically. The endeavor is not difficult, recognizing your own Nature is.

87

欲學果與誠

YU XUE GUO YU CHENG

to desire, to learn, determined, and, sincere
to desire to learn, determined and sincere

If you want to learn, then you must be determined and sincere.

You must immerse yourself in that which you want to learn. Study the history, learn about the teachers, see how your system differs from others. This opens your consciousness to the entire system and to all who have contributed to it. My teacher would say that the student who doesn't want to put in the effort has the heart and mind of a tourist.

88

久恆與智慧

JIU HENG YU ZHI HUI

a long time, persevering, and, wisdom, intelligence
a long time persevering, and, wisdom, intelligence

Your success depends upon tireless perseverance as well as wisdom and intelligence.

What you learn has to blend with your everyday life. Too much practice will take you over the edge. I've been there. Harmony and Balance, emblazon those words upon the walls of your consciousness. Tireless perseverance should be mitigated by wisdom and intelligence. Always seek the dynamically relaxed place in your practice so that in the stillness you can be guided by the wisdom from within.

89

華嶽希夷門

HUA YUE XI YI MEN

Hua Yue, Xiyi, a sect
The sect of [Ch'ên] Xiyi of Hua Yue.

Liuhebafa has been carried on by the disciples of Chen Xiyi of Mount Hua.

Li Dongfeng learned the system with the help of the monks and hermits who lived on the sacred western mountain, Hua Shan. After Li left Mount Hua, he returned to Mount Yun where he taught a small group of Daoists. From that small group, we can trace the lineage of Liuhebafa to the present day.

90

力行最為貴

LI XING ZUI WEI GUI

strength, to act, exceedingly, to be, to hold in honor
act with exceeding effort, to be held in honor

You should strive to be an example of your Art.

The practice of Liuhebafa gives you the opportunity to rise to the heights of excellence in the martial arts. You should honor and respect the masters who have gone before and passed down this most excellent method to you. It is only right and fitting that you strive to be a positive example to others and represent your art with the highest morals and ethics.

91

神意要集中

SHEN YI YAO JI ZHONG

spirit, the will, necessary, to gather together, middle
spirit and the will, necessary to gather together, middle

It is essential that spirit and intent come together at the center within.

Spirit is that energy from which all things are made. There is no place that it is not. An intention, desire, or goal that is impressed upon or placed into this energy will be manifested if that intention, desire, or goal is contemplated or dwelled upon at the stillpoint within. The Six Combinations of Liuhebafa demonstrate how energy becomes matter and how matter returns to energy. The secret that the masters reveal is that you can work with this energy or underlying Life Force consciously. Your link to the Source is through gratitude and service. There is nothing within the Life Force that is withheld from you.

92

推動輪轉器

TUI DONG LUN ZHUAN QI

to push, to move, to revolve, to turn, implements
to motivate, to rotate, implements

Your intention and spirit together move all parts of the body as one unit.

Body, Heart/Mind, Will/Intent, *Qi*, and Spirit combine into one unity that has the characteristics of being still, non-resistant, and deliberate. So, when one thing moves, everything moves. The hand should not move without the whole body moving. From the soles of your feet to the top of your head, all is in harmony.

Boxing requires action, but first you must be internally still.

Meeting an opponent requires force, but first you are internally non-resistant.

Combat requires speed, but first you are deliberate.

93

一觸力即發

Yi Chu Li Ji Fa

one, to touch, strength, immediately, to issue
once touched, strength, immediately issued

The moment you are touched your strength immediately issues.

Your first step in specific training to issue energy is to learn the Main Form. After you have mastered the movements, you use your Creative Imagination. While practicing the form, you imagine the energy issuing from your bones and joints. You then practice issuing energy as you encounter an imaginary opponent. This kind of practice opens the energy gates so that when you need the power it will flow immediately.

94

使敵難迴避

SHI DI NAN BI

to cause, opponent, difficult, to turn around, to evade
to cause the opponent, difficult, to turn around to escape

Your skill makes it difficult for your opponent to move or escape.

Through training you become perceptive, receptive, and sensitive. With practice, you first learn to feel another's energy so that you can neutralize it and dispatch them. The second level is more subtle in that your energy can discharge into someone who simply brushes you or you can withdraw all of his or her strength by a light touch. The third is a profound neutralizing of gravitational fields, and is rarely, if ever, seen these days. Such applications confuses and overcomes your opponent because every way he turns, there you are adhering to him. There is no getting rid of you.

95

欲鬆似非鬆

YU SONG SI FEI SONG

to desire, to relax, resembling, without, to relax
to desire to relax, resembling, without relaxing

You appear calm and relaxed; but like a cat, you are always ready.

Through the methods of Liuhebafa you will learn how to dynamically relax. Watch a cat. The cat is relaxing in the sun and has the appearance of being asleep but the slightest noise and the cat is up and ready.

If that sleeping cat is pounced by another cat, you will see the instantaneous release of great power. You can do this. Relaxation and courage must coexist within you; so, the key here is to be without fear. When you are without fear, you can be calm. From the calm state, your inner power can issue without hesitation.

96

欲緊未著力

YU JIN WEI ZHUO LI

to desire, tense, not, to see, brute strength
to desire tension, not to see, brute strength

You may want to show tension but do not show your raw strength.

This Secret emphasizes the Methods of Feature and Conceal. Through Feature you can mislead your opponent by giving them the appearance of being tense and afraid. This allows them to be over confident and misjudge the situation. Then, when they have committed to their attack, you reveal your true power that you have concealed behind the image of temerity. Surprise is a valuable tool in combat. Again, *The Art of War* is a primer for your approach to combat and life.

97

運使求均衡

YUN SHI QIU JUN HENG

to revolve, to employ, to seek after, equally,
to balance
employ revolving, to seek after, equally balanced

To attain equal and even balance make all of your movements circular.

In Liuhebafa foundation training, circular movement is used first in the joints, and then is applied throughout your body. You cannot extend your movement circularly unless you have made small circles inwardly. This also relates to letting your energy circulate naturally to attain a balanced energy state. Often in training, you might try too hard to do a movement or technique; this use of the will overtaxes the spleen which will take energy from your bones and kidneys thus weakening the body. Always, therefore, seek the neutral point so that the energy can flow freely in its natural courses.

98

螺旋循環氣

LUO XUAN XUN HUAN QI

spiral, to revolve, to follow, ring, qi
spiral revolves, to follow, a circle of qi

Your *qi* follows circularly in a revolving spiral.

Your energy spirals down from the top of your head to your feet, heaven to earth and vice versa. By training to move in circles, you harmonize with this circular and rotational flow of energy. This is the way energy is compressed and released (issued). This fluid and spiral-like issuing of energy is a hallmark of Liuhebafa.

99

遇敵勿惶張

YU DI WU HUANG QI

to meet, opponent, do not, agitated, fear
to meet the opponent, do not, fearful or agitated

When encountering the opponent do not be fearful or agitated.

Long practice can make your body as hard as stone, as resilient as a steel spring, and as fluid as water; but that alone will not give you an assurance of your skills. It is only through your inner training where you will have met your true fears and dissolved them. Fear, anger, lack of confidence are dissolved in the stillness in which you hold the image of the person you want to be, a person who is strong and courageous. Impress this image of yourself on the energy of the Life Force and you will not be fearful or agitated when you face an opponent.

100

開合收與放

KAI HE SHOU YU FANG

to open, to close, to collect, and, to release
to open and close, to collect and release

Use the movements of Closing and Opening
to Gather and Release your inner power.

Stretch (Open) and Contract (Close) your waist to exert strength. All movement proceeds from your center. Through the pumping action of opening and closing, you learn how to effectively issue strength through any part of your body. First, however, you must sink all of your weight and energy into the soles of your feet. This takes a lot of dedicated practice time. Once settled in your feet, the energy bubbles back up to the solar plexus where it can be released as force through the movement of your center.

The term "Open and Close" also carries the connotation of being "Empty and Full". The pulling in action of *closing* will gather energy as if you were a sponge soaking up water. The outflow of *open* will release or radiate energy from every pore outward like heat from a wood stove.

After you get the feel of the inflow and outflow of energy, you train to get the energy to issue from a single point directed by your attention. One way to do this is to focus your attention on the flame of a candle. Raise your arm and point your hand towards the flame. First, make the flame go away from you and then come back toward you. After some success at that, work to extinguish the candle flame. You will be amazed at the relative ease of this if you are aligned, relaxed and breathing naturally.

101

見形尋破綻

JIAN XING XUN PO ZHAN

to observe, form, to seek, to break, a hint
observe the form, to seek, a hint of a break

Carefully observe your form to seek out any weak point.

If there is a weak point in your skills, an experienced opponent may find it. Your form is an expression of your understanding of the movement of energy and your cooperation with it. Constantly practice, there is always another step to take.

102

絲毫不相讓

SI HAO BU XIANG RANG

small, hair, not, mutual, to yield
the smallest hair, non reciprocal, to yield

Do not yield even the smallest hair.

It is said that skilled Xingyi boxers would face each other for hours to perceive an opening. This required much training, strength, stamina, and discipline. You must train diligently to gain this kind of skill; so that when you go out to meet your opponent, you can have the discipline to conceal your true ability.

103

腕肘肩胯膝

Wan Zhou Jian Kua Xi

wrist, elbow, shoulder, space between the legs, knee
wrists, elbows, shoulders, space between the legs, and knees.

Maintain the circles in your wrists, elbows, shoulders, hips, and knees.

Work to combine or unify these nine joints into one coherent unity to conceal the *qi* in the marrow of your bones. Through patient and calm practice of foundation and the Main Form, you learn to circle the energy through these areas to maintain a settled, confident quality in your body. This confidence helps you to face the enemy.

104

足踏手腳齊

Zu Ta Shou Jiao Qi

foot, to walk, hand, leg, together
the feet walk, hands and legs, together

When you take a step your hands move correspondingly.

Explore the depth of Liuhebafa. Consider the reasoning behind the movements. Why do you move the way you do? Why does the energy move up from the sole of your foot to issue out of your hand? The answer can be found in an examination of the unified five hearts. The five hearts are the centers of the two feet, the center of the two palms, and the center of the top of the head. By placing your attention on the five hearts, you can connect with the collective consciousness of the Liuhebafa system.

The collective consciousness of the system is the repository of all knowledge and experience of previous Liuhebafa masters over the centuries. This knowledge and experience flows out of a morphic field when we have the acceptance of it. So, when you step forward, the entire body of knowledge and understanding steps with you. And this is true of any movement you do.

To access this morphic field, you can use either a standing or sitting contemplation posture. When you have settled into your posture, set your intention to access the collective consciousness of Liuhebafa. Begin by placing your attention on the centers of your two feet (Well of the Bubbling Springs). Next, move your attention to the centers of your two palms (Labored Palace). Finally, place your attention on the top of your head (Mount Kunlun). Let the energy rise from your feet to your palms and then to the top of your head. Feel the energy rise just above your head, then sweep your immediate area 360 degrees around you like radar. Then calmly listen. You may hear any number of sounds such as the sound of distant drums or the tinkling of bells. When you hear the sound, follow it to its origin. It will lead you to the thing you seek.

105

節節力貫串

JIE JIE LI GUAN CHUAN

joint, joint, strength, to go through,
to string together
joints, strength, to go through, to string together

When all your joints are joined or connected the inner strength moves through them.

Through the practice of the foundation methods of Liuhebafa, you can connect all your joints. It is your intention, however, that moves the energy through the marrow. Review the Secrets listed below:

14. The entire body is elastic and spring-like.

68. The power flows through the five terminals and nine joints.

33. Just as strength is stored in the curve of a bow, so do you store strength in the curves of your body.

34. Issue your strength like an arrow, direct, and straight.

91. It is essential that spirit and intent come together at the center within.

92. Your intention and spirit together move all parts of the body as one unit.

100. Use the movements of Closing and Opening to gather and release your inner power.

105. When all your joints are joined or connected the inner strength moves through them.

106. When you are trained there will be no cracks in your armor.

120. Connecting the joints makes the storage of strength tangible or real.

121. Stretching your joints activates and enlivens the blood vessels.

106

處處無乘隙

CHU CHU WU CHENG XI

place, place, without, take advantage of, a crack
everywhere, without, take advantage of a crack

When you are trained, there will be no cracks in your armor.

By cultivating circular movements that follow the spiraling energy and by unifying body, mind, and spirit, you will go where you will with nothing to fear.

Follow the eight methods:

Qi works internally concentrated by spirit.

Bone conceals the internal force.

Feature is fluid and continuous.

Listen, Follow, Receive, and Neutralize an attack.

Lift your attention above your head.
Return hastens the power and speed of your internal force.
Restrain your mind to be calm.
Conceal your true power.

107

呼吸細綿綿

HU XI XI MIAN MIAN

to exhale, to inhale, fine, soft or continuous,
soft or continuous
to breathe, fine, soft and continuous

When inhaling and exhaling, your breath is fine, soft, and continuous.

The finest silk thread is pulled from a cocoon carefully and continuously. Your breathing reflects the movement of energy in your body. If your breathing is strained or shallow, this is the way the energy flows. With training, your breathing becomes regular and softly balanced so that your energy moves freely throughout your body.

108

升降緩而急

SHENG JIANG HUAN ER JI

to ascend, to descend, slow, yet, hurried
to ascend and descend, slow and yet hurried

Whether your movement is slow or fast, your breathing will rise and fall naturally.

Just as you train all movement to flow from your center, teach your movements to follow your breath. Thus, with time, your breathing becomes deeper, stronger, and more natural.

We don't advocate any particular method of breathing except that it be natural. With time and dynamically relaxed practice, you will naturally begin to breathe from your center. Thus your breathing can support the needs of any activity without strain.

109

得法可應變

DE FA KE YING BIAN

to acquire, method, can, to respond, to change
to acquire this method, can respond to change

When this [breathing] method is acquired, you can respond to any change.

When you have mastered Natural Breathing, you have acquired the calm state. You can now issue force effortlessly. Every movement is coordinated and in harmony. There is nothing that will restrict the free flow of energy. You have attained the neutral state. You can adapt to any and all conditions and changes.

110

有術方為奇

YOU SHU FANG WEI QI

to have, art, method, to be, remarkable
to have, art and method, is to be rare

To have both the art [wisdom] and its methods [techniques] is rare.

Some people count over seven hundred techniques in the Main Form. However, don't become infatuated with techniques because the heart of the system is actually without technique. Your ability to truly express this art comes only from knowingness, not from knowledge.

111

法術二而一

FA SHU ER ER YI

method, art, two, and yet, one
method and art, two and yet one

Method and art are two and yet one.

In Liuhebafa, your understanding of Life is expressed as the unity of understanding and the method through which it is expressed.

There is method and art in each of the three phases of Liuhebafa: Earth, Man, and Heaven.

The **Earth phase** teaches advanced survival skills.

The **Man phase** teaches the student to look at others with equanimity and compassion.

The **Heaven phase** opens the heart and shows the way to the Original Source, our True Home.

112

缺一不能立

QUE YI BU NENG LI

a weakness, one, not, to be able, to stand
one weakness, unable to stand

If there is but a single weakness you will not be able to withstand an opponent.

A famous Taiji fighter was challenged. Although he 'won' the fight, the sleeve of his coat was torn. When his father saw this, he said that the skill used was not Taiji. So it is in Liuhebafa, our purpose is to maintain harmony not to use technique to enforce our will and strength on others. Fighting to force your will on others will eventually have to be balanced; this follows the law of cause and effect.

113

兩手輕輕起

LIANG SHOU QING QING QI

both, hands, light, light, to raise
both hands, lightly, to raise

Raise both hands lightly.

Arm strength is not used to raise your arms. Let them float up. The impetus for this movement comes from the opening and closing of the scapula. This opening and closing pumps the energy out to your arms to raise and lower them. Of course this movement is preparatory to issuing force.

114

曲伸無斷續

QU SHEN WU DUAN XU

bent, to stretch out, without, to interrupt, continuous
bent, to stretch out, without interruption, continuous

Continuously bend and stretch without interruption.

Circularity is the key here. The bending and stretching is fluid, connected movement in curves. You see this kind of movement in a graceful dancer. Get video recordings of famous martial artists and dancers and watch their movement, then try to copy it. Get the idea of it into your movement. You will be surprised how quickly your movement will soften and become more fluid. If you have the idea (picture) in your mind, you will be far ahead of the person just doing rote movement.

115

轉移有曲折

ZHUAN YI YOU QU ZHE

to turn, to shift, to have, bent, to bend
to turn and shift, to have, bent around

All your turning and shifting follows curves.

Turning and bending in the external methods is linear, but the internal method favors the movement of nature that always follows curves. In the external it is force against force, head on. The internal is circular and meets the attack with softness with yielding that guides the hard energy into the void.

The external is obvious; the internal is concealed with its force deep within the marrow of the bones where it is not obvious. Relaxation is a requisite to circularity. The internal method must come out of being calm and settled at the stillpoint within. Otherwise, the so-called internal practice will be soft external kung fu.

116

形似遊龍戲

XING SI YOU LONG XI

form, to resemble, to roam, dragon, to play
form resembles, to roam, dragon at play

The form movements resemble a roaming dragon at play.

The dragon undulates and coils from its center. But the intent of the dragon is hidden by the playful, light-hearted nature of the movement.

Just so, your power must coil and undulate from the solar plexus as you practice the form. Keep your heart and mind on your heart's desire as you practice so that the movements will appear light and playful.

117

縱橫起與伏

Zong Heng Qi Yu Fu

vertical, horizontal, to rise, and, to prostrate
vertically, horizontally, rising, and prostrate

Your movement can rise up vertically or be flat on the ground.

Like water, you can rise to the heights or seek the lowest places. There is no limit to the type of movement or technique that you can do. One of Liuhebafa's favorite animals is the dragon. You can emulate the dragon while practicing the Main Form. Like the dragon you can undulate up or down or turn back powerfully upon yourself. The light and playful way in which you do these difficult movements deceptively hides the power within.

118

陰陽運行數

YIN YANG YUN XING SHU

Yin, Yang, to revolve, to travel, an art
Yin and Yang, travel back and forth, an art

The movement back and forth between *Yin* and *Yang* is an art.

In your study of cause and effect, you see that one becomes the other. You find that you can intercept a strong attack with soft energy and conversely repel a soft attack with hard energy. Liuhebafa's emphasis on moving in circles, internally and externally, aids in expressing and understanding the laws of polarity.

In combat, you must strive to maintain unity and which side of duality you utilize will depend totally on the situation. Moving seamlessly back and forth between the two is an art.

119

意動氣相隨

QI DONG QI XIANG SUI

intent, to move, qi, mutually, to follow
intent moves, qi, follows immediately after

Where the Mind (Intent) goes the *qi* immediately follows.

This is true whether for good or for ill. Be careful where or on what you place your attention.

120

關節含蓄力

GUAN JIE HAN XU LI

to connect, joints, to embody, to store, strength
connect joints, to embody, to store strength

Connecting the joints makes the storage of strength tangible or real.

The *qi* that has been compacted into your bone marrow through the training methods of Liuhebafa flows out through the joints. Your joints act like step up transformers. When your joints are strung together or connected, the energy or power in the body becomes easily recognizable to your senses, i.e., audible, perceptible, noticeable; therefore obvious, evident, plain, and clear to the mind.

121

舒筋活血脈

SHU JIN HUO XUE MAI

to stretch out, joints, active, blood, veins or arteries
to stretch out the joints, activate, blood vessels

Stretching your joints activates and enlivens the blood vessels.

When you stretch your joints and ligaments together, your body becomes unified, connected. Your energy can then flow unimpeded outward into your whole body, into the extremities. This will enhance the outflow and inflow pulse of blood from your heart. It is said that the *qi* pulls the blood like the moon pulls the tides.

122

榮衛得適宜

Rong Wei De Shi Yi

blood, to protect, to attain, to succeed, fitting
to protect the blood, to attain,
to succeed in being fit

By protecting your blood [with *qi*], you will attain health and succeed in being fit.

The Chinese classics say that reinforcing your blood, breath, and bone are fundamental to good health. All of your Liuhebafa stretching and breathing exercises strengthen your blood, breath, and bone with life-giving *qi*. *Qi* flowing throughout your body pulls the oxygenated blood into and through the organs to purify your whole system. Your purified system then becomes able to move ever more *qi* and blood that restores and maintains your health. You must be fit to face an opponent.

123 & 124

一吸氣便提

YI XI QI BIAN TI

one, inhale, qi, then, to raise
one inhale, qi then rises

氣下可歸臍

QI XIA KE GUI QI

qi, to descend, can, return, navel
qi descends, can return to the navel

When you inhale the *qi* rises [to the top of the head], then descends to return to the *dantien* [abdomen].

This is the natural rise and fall of the energy in your body and describes the microcosmic circuit of energy. In the microcosmic circuit, as you breathe in, the energy is pulled from your abdomen down to the base of your spine, up the spine, across the top of your head and then returns to your abdomen by moving down over your forehead, through the roof of your mouth, on down your throat, through your stomach to your abdomen.

The above is considered the most common pathway through this circuit. However, there are other ways that the energy may travel which are natural from individual to individual. The methods of Liuhebafa do not dictate a particular pattern. The methods you use enhance the natural flow of energy through the body so that it will issue when needed, naturally.

125

一提氣便咽

YI TI QI BIAN YAN

one, to raise, qi, to use, to swallow
one, to raise the qi, use swallowing

Once the *qi* rises, swallow on its return to the *dantien*.

One of the initial exercises you do involves consciously moving or following the movement of the energy through the microcosmic orbit. This orbit runs from the top of your head down the front of your body to your coccyx and back up again following your spine. As the energy passes through the roof of your mouth and into your tongue, the swallowing of your saliva aids in the physical awareness of the movement of this energy. Martially, this practice will help to keep you from getting 'cotton mouth' when you get into a tense situation. Thereby helping you maintain your center.

The esoteric side suggests that by swallowing your breath (or nectar) of heaven, you can gain enlightenment.

126

水火得相見

SHUI HUO DE XIANG JIAN

water, fire, succeed, mutual, to see
water and fire, succeed, to meet

Fire from above and Water from below meet harmoniously.

Fire (energy) and Water (essence) should be in balance to maintain a harmony in your body. If there is too much Fire or too much Water, your organs will be affected. Symptoms of dryness or dampness, heat or coolness are results of an unbalanced mental state or improper practices. Proper practice ensures that your organs will be stimulated and toned by this work. Before you begin any practice, take contemplative time to still the internal dialogue and calm your mind; this will help bring inner physical harmony to all your organs.

127

精研內外功

JING YAN NEI WAI GONG

the essence of, to investigate thoroughly, internal, external, achievement
thoroughly investigate the essence of, internal, external, achievement

A complete investigation is necessary to thoroughly understand the essence of this achievement [kung fu] that is both internal and external.

One year, Li Zhong offered a weekend seminar on the subtleties of the Main Form. One of the students who was helping with the arrangements asked if the attendees would receive a certificate when they finished the weekend course. He laughed and said, "A piece of paper cannot say what you know". He never gave certificates or letters attesting to ability or proficiency. His point of view is that you should make this a life-long experiment to examine and prove the truths of this system to yourself.

This system has a Main Form, but it is not form driven. It is driven by Intention, which begins internally and manifests externally. This system is a treasure that must be sought. *The Five Character Secrets* is the treasure map.

128

心虛腹要實

XIN XU FU YAO SHI

the mind (heart), empty, abdomen, necessary, solid
the mind (heart), is empty, abdomen necessary to be solid

Empty your Mind (Heart) and reinforce your abdomen [to achieve enlightenment].

This Secret follows the old saying that you must keep your head in heaven and your feet upon the earth. One of the ways you connect with the earth is through your rooting techniques through which you build your foundation in your lower body (waist downward). Once you have the physical stamina to walk, row, or stand then the inner channels open and the energy flows up from the well of the bubbling springs (kidney meridian) to the *dantien* located in the abdomen. With your connection firmly reinforced to the earth, you can then begin to open your Heart Center to move your consciousness and attention upward through your Third Eye and Crown Chakra to the different levels or dimensions of heaven to achieve enlightenment.

129

牽然取其勢

QIAN RAN QU QI SHI

to pull, certainly, to take hold of, his, circumstance
pulling, to take hold of, his circumstances

Seize your opportunity to control the situation.

As you become more aware, you see that there are opportunities all around us; all it takes is an attitude of acceptance and gratitude. Unfortunately, when you get into a bad spot and your attitude sours, opportunities seem to disappear or dissolve in front of you. This is sort of like painting yourself into a corner, and you just have to wait until the paint dries.

It is good to be courageous and take the chance on an opportunity and not over analyze it. You can analyze an opportunity away. It is said that the first time an opportunity comes it is presented as a gold cup. If you don't take it, it comes around again as a silver cup. If you don't take it, it comes around as an iron cup. Get it? Be bold and adventuresome and take the golden opportunity when it comes.

130

首尾不相離

SHOU WEI BU XIANG LI

head, tail, not, mutually, to separate
head and tail, not mutually to separate

The beginning and ending are inseparable.

Nothing in this world lasts forever. When something is begun, that it will have to end is a certainty. Birth and Death go together. It is the Life in between that is important, and what you do with it. So, dream of what you want and want to become. See it as a reality. Touch it, smell it, taste it, listen to it. This where you set your goal or intention, at the beginning. If you set the beginning, the ending or the manifesting of what you want is already determined by your desire. This how the beginning and ending are inseparable or the same.

131

奇正得相宜

QI ZHENG DE XIANG YI

strange, orthodox, to attain, mutual, is necessary
strange, orthodox, is necessary to attain mutual

Opposites (ordinary/extraordinary) are necessary to achieve a mutual function.

Opposites, Yin and Yang, flow one into the other. You simply cannot exist in the worlds of matter without the one or the other. Inner and outer, hard and soft become one because you, from the neutral point of view, see them coming together and blending to produce a mutual function. As you learn to harmonize with these 'energies', you can stir them around to confuse and confound your opponent.

132

動靜隨心欲

DONG JING SUI XIN YU

to move, to be still, to follow, mind (heart), to desire
in movement and in stillness, follow, the heart's desire

In movement and in stillness, follow your heart's desire.

Throughout *The Five Character Secrets of Li Dongfeng*, you have had repeated to you over and over again in one form or another that you, through your thoughts, can change your world into whatever you wish. Some will take this work to heart and manifest a devastatingly deadly fighting system. Others will find their way to health and well-being. And yet others, who pursue the hidden truths, will use these secrets to follow the way to the Source.

What do you want? Place your attention (intention) on it and hold it there with all the discipline you can muster. You will find that where the mind goes the energy follows. The energy needs your thoughts as a mold to fulfill your inner desires and dreams. Today's thoughts and desires are tomorrow's conditions. So, listen to your Inner Voice (in stillness and movement) and do what you truly want to do. Creatively manifesting your heart's desire is completely up to you.

133 & 134

龘成五字訣

CU CHENG WU ZI JUE

coarse, to complete, Five Character Secrets
coarse completion, Five Character Secrets

後學莫輕視

HOU XUE MO QING SHI

afterwards, to study, do not, lightly, to inspect
to study afterwards, do not, to inspect lightly

This ends the Five Character Secrets of Li Dongfeng. Take care to study it carefully and do not take it lightly.

The
Five
Character
Secrets

1. MIND/INTENT IS THE BASIS OF METHODLESSNESS.

心意本無法

2. USE THE METHOD OF EMPTINESS.

有法是虛無

3. EMPTINESS IS USED TO ACQUIRE THE NATURAL STATE.

虛無得自然

4. TO BE WITHOUT A METHOD IS UNFORGIVABLE.

無法不容恕

5. RELAX IN ORDER TO FILL EVERYWHERE.

放之彌六合

6. WRAP UP HEAVEN AND EARTH WHICH ARE SMALL.

包羅小天地

7. THE BUDDHISTS EXPRESS THEIR PERCEPTION OF THE NATURAL STATE WITH A CIRCLE.

釋家為覺圓

8. THE DAOISTS SPEAK OF LEAVING NOTHING BEHIND.

道家說無遺

9. HAVING FEATURE, SEEK AFTERWARD THE
FEATURELESS.

有象求無象

10. THERE IS NO SET TIME LIMIT IN ACHIEVING THE
NATURAL STATE OF BEING.

不期自然至

11. IF YOU WANT TO LEARN THE INTERNAL ACHIEVE-
MENT OF MIND/INTENT.

要學心意功

12. THEN YOU MUST FIRST BEGIN TO FOLLOW THE
EIGHT METHODS.

先從八法起

13. CULTIVATE THE TEMPERAMENT OF
RIGHTEOUSNESS.

養我浩然氣

14. THE ENTIRE BODY IS COMPLETELY ELASTIC AND
SPRING-LIKE.

遍身皆彈力

15. THE BEGINNING IS EVIDENT BUT NOT THE ENDING.

見首不見尾

16. EXPRESS NEITHER FEATURE NOR INTENT.

無象亦無意

17. RECEIVE AND RELEASE WITHOUT SHOWING FORM.

收放勿露形

18. YOUR RELAXING OR TENSING IS NECESSARILY SELF-CONTROLLED.

鬆緊要自主

19. IT IS NECESSARY TO BE CALM FOR A PROPER RESPONSE TO AN ATTACK.

策應宜守默

20. NEITHER INCLINE NOR LEAN, REMAIN STRAIGHT IN YOUR STANCE.

不偏亦不倚

21. YOU APPEAR UNABLE, EVEN WHEN YOU ARE ABLE.

視不能如能

22. IF INEXPERIENCED, DO NOT ENGAGE THE OPPONENT.

生疏莫臨敵

23. EVEN DURING MOVEMENT, USE YOUR ENERGY TO MAINTAIN A FIRM ROOT.

動時把得固

24. WHEN YOU ISSUE ENERGY (STRIKE), DO NOT OVEREXTEND YOURSELF TO YOUR OPPONENT.

一發未得人

25. LOOK FOR THE RIGHT TIME (OPPORTUNITY) TO MAKE YOUR MOVE (ATTACK).

審機得其勢

26. PROTECT YOURSELF AND TAKE ADVANTAGE OF THE OPPONENT BY STRIKING FIRST.

乘敵擊與顧

27. IN A CONFRONTATION, YOU MAY SEE HARDNESS IN THE STRENGTH OF OTHERS.

剛在他力前

28. YOUR SOFTNESS WILL TAKE ADVANTAGE OF YOUR OPPONENT'S (HARD) STRENGTH BY LEADING IT INTO EMPTINESS.

柔乘他力後

29. WHEN HE RUSHES TO ATTACK, I AM QUIET AND
CALMLY WAIT.

彼忙我静待

30. YOU CONTROL THE CONFRONTATION, YOU DECIDE
WHEN TO ATTACK OR DEFEND.

攻守任君鬥

31. METHODICALLY AND QUICKLY OVERCOME YOUR
OPPONENT.

步步佔先機

32. KEEP YOUR AWARENESS (ATTENTION) ON THE BUSI-
NESS AT HAND.

時時要留意

33. JUST AS STRENGTH IS STORED IN THE CURVE OF A
BOW, SO DO YOU STORE STRENGTH IN THE CURVES
OF YOUR BODY.

蓄勁如弓圓

34. ISSUE YOUR STRENGTH LIKE AN ARROW, DIRECT
AND STRAIGHT.

發勁似箭直

35. YOU MUST THOROUGHLY UNDERSTAND THE LAW OF OPPOSITES (YIN/YANG).

悟透陰陽理

36. HARD AND SOFT COME TOGETHER TO MUTUALLY BLEND.

剛柔互參就

37. COORDINATE YOUR BREATH FOR THE QUALITIES OF WATER AND FIRE TO EXCHANGE.

調息坎離交

38. NO MATTER WHETHER YOUR BREATHING IS UP, DOWN, OR IN THE MIDDLE, THE CHI WILL BE SMOOTH AND HARMONIOUS.

上下中和氣

39. MAINTAIN THE QUIETNESS AND CALMNESS OF A BUDDHIST IN REPOSE.

守默為臥禪

40. MOVE LIKE A DRAGON RISING FROM HIBERNATION.

動似蟄龍起

41. WITHIN THE SPIRIT OF EMPTINESS IS EMBODIED THE SUBSTANTIAL.

虛靈含有物

42. As you hasten to become profoundly obscure (Spirit of Emptiness).

窈窈冥冥趣

43. You will be able to suddenly express or suddenly conceal (your internal force).

忽隱又忽現

44. Regard every breath you take as being natural.

息息任自然

45. Evade and avoid the heavy strength (attack) of an opponent.

避免敵重力

46. You are responsible for every action.

原來自我始

47. Make the difference between double and single [weightedness] clear.

雙單可分明

48. Yin and Yang manifest in both the empty and solid.

陰陽見虛實

49. EMPTINESS CAN BE USED TO LEAD AN OPPONENT TO FALL INTO A VOID.

虛引敵落空

50. IT IS DESIROUS TO QUICKLY CHANGE BETWEEN RECEIVING ENERGY AND RELEASING ENERGY.

欲收放更急

51. BOTH LEGS SHOULD RESEMBLE THE CURVE OF A BOW.

兩腿似弓彎

52. STRETCH (OPEN) AND CONTRACT (CLOSE) THE WAIST TO EXERT STRENGTH.

伸縮腰著力

53. THE BACK AND ARMS ARE ROUNDED INTO A CIRCULAR EMBRACE.

脊臂須環抱

54. MIXING THE ORIGINAL QI IS ALWAYS FROM WITHIN (INTERNAL TO EXTERNAL).

內外混元氣

55. A WAY TO HALT WANDERING THOUGHTS SO THAT YOU CAN FOCUS.

息念要集神

56. IS TO ACT AS IF YOU ARE FACING A GREAT AND
FAMOUS FIGHTER.

彷佛臨大敵

57. BRIGHT AND FULL OF LIFE, YOUR EYES MOVE LIKE
LIGHTNING.

目光如電流

58. YOUR HIGHER AWARENESS ENCOMPASSES 360
DEGREES.

精神顧四隅

59. KEEP 40% IN THE FRONT LEG
AND 60% IN THE REAR LEG.

前四後佔六

60. YOUR HAND STRENGTH LIES 30% FORWARD AND
70% BACK TOWARD THE BODY.

掌握三與七

61. WHEN YOU DO THE FORM, MOVE LIKE YOU ARE
SWIMMING IN WATER.

形動如浴水

62. MOVE LIKE CLOUDS AND MISTS CLEARING IN THE
SKY,

若履雲霧霽

63. AS YOU FLOAT GRACEFULLY TO GREET AN IMMORTAL IN THE CLOUDS.

飄飄呼欲仙

64. YOU WILL FIND THE MAJESTIC GREATNESS IN PURE EMPTINESS.

浩浩乎清虛

65. YOUR CREATIVE IMAGINATION (INTENT) MOVES LIKE A FEARSOME TIGER.

意動似懼虎

66. YOUR QI MOVES CALMLY LIKE A GENTLE YOUNG LADY.

氣動如處子

67. AS SOON AS THE OPPONENT MOVES TO ATTACK, HE WILL IMMEDIATELY BE KNOCKED DOWN.

犯者敵即仆

68. THE POWER FLOWS THROUGH THE FIVE TERMINALS AND NINE JOINTS.

五總九節力

69. IF YOU WANT TO LEARN AND UNDERSTAND, YOU MUST HAVE PERSEVERANCE.

欲學持有恆

70. YOU MUST ADVANCE INTO THE HALL BEFORE YOU CAN ENTER THE (MASTER'S) CHAMBER.

升堂可入室

71. YOUR APPEARANCE OF HAVING OR NOT HAVING INNER FORCE WILL BE DISPLAYED OR CONCEALED NATURALLY.

顯隱無與有

72. HAVE A SPIRIT OF SKEPTICISM AS YOU SEEK TO INVESTIGATE THE TRUTH.

疑神尋真諦

73. THIS WONDERFUL METHOD (LIUHEBAFA) COMBINES ALL MOVEMENT HARMONIOUSLY.

妙法有和合

74. SEPARATE THE SPIRIT WITH EMPTINESS AND SOLITUDE.

離神空虛寂

75. THE WAY TO THESE PRINCIPLES IS EXTREMELY FINE AND SUBTLE.

拳拳得服膺

76. IT IS WISE TO KEEP THE SECRETS YOU ATTAIN TO YOURSELF.

道理極細微

77. WHEN YOU ARE MOVING DESIRE TO APPEAR AS THOUGH YOU ARE NOT MOVING.

欲動似非動

78. WITHIN THE CENTER OF YOUR STILLNESS, MAINTAIN YOUR INTENT.

静中還有意

79. CEASE WANDERING THOUGHTS AND THE FLOW OF YOUR QI WILL BECOME CALM AND EVEN.

息念氣自平

80. SILENTLY MAINTAIN THE GREAT EMPTINESS.

默默守太虛

81. THE FIRST STEP IN LEARNING THIS SYSTEM IS BUILDING A FIRM FOUNDATION.

元根築基法

82. COLLECT YOUR PEARLS AND JADE, BUT KEEP THEM ALL CONCEALED.

蘊藏皆珠玉

83. LIUHEBAFA IS SAID TO BE BOTH DIFFICULT AND NOT DIFFICULT.

說難亦非難

84. THINGS USUALLY AREN'T AS EASY AS THEY FIRST APPEAR.

看易本非易

85. IN ANY ENDEAVOR, YOU MUST HAVE THE DETERMINATION TO FINISH AND SUCCEED.

有志事竟成

86. IN THIS WORLD, THERE IS NO ENDEAVOR THAT IS DIFFICULT.

世間無難事

87. IF YOU WANT TO LEARN, THEN YOU MUST BE DETERMINED AND SINCERE.

欲學果與誠

88. YOUR SUCCESS DEPENDS UPON TIRELESS PERSEVERANCE AS WELL AS WISDOM AND INTELLIGENCE.

久恆與智慧

89. LIUHEBAFA HAS BEEN CARRIED ON BY THE DISCIPLES OF CHEN XIYI OF MOUNT HUA.

華嶽希夷門

90. YOU SHOULD STRIVE TO BE AN EXAMPLE OF YOUR ART.

力行最為貴

91. IT IS ESSENTIAL THAT SPIRIT AND INTENT COME TOGETHER AT THE CENTER WITHIN.

神意要集中

92. YOUR INTENTION AND SPIRIT TOGETHER MOVE ALL PARTS OF THE BODY AS ONE UNIT.

推動輪轉器

93. THE MOMENT YOU ARE TOUCHED YOUR STRENGTH IMMEDIATELY ISSUES.

一觸力即發

94. YOUR SKILL MAKES IT DIFFICULT FOR YOUR OPPONENT TO MOVE OR ESCAPE.

使敵難迴避

95. YOU APPEAR CALM AND RELAXED; BUT LIKE A CAT, YOU ARE ALWAYS READY.

欲鬆似非鬆

96. YOU MAY WANT TO SHOW TENSION BUT DO NOT SHOW YOUR RAW STRENGTH.

欲緊未著力

97. TO ATTAIN EQUAL AND EVEN BALANCE MAKE ALL OF YOUR MOVEMENTS CIRCULAR.

運使求均衡

98. YOUR QI FOLLOWS CIRCULARLY IN A REVOLVING SPIRAL.

螺旋循環氣

99. WHEN ENCOUNTERING THE OPPONENT DO NOT BE FEARFUL OR AGITATED.

遇敵勿惶張

100. USE THE MOVEMENTS OF CLOSING AND OPENING TO GATHER AND RELEASE YOUR INNER POWER.

開合收與放

101. CAREFULLY OBSERVE YOUR FORM TO SEEK OUT ANY WEAK POINT.

見形尋破綻

102. DO NOT YIELD EVEN THE SMALLEST HAIR.

絲毫不相讓

103. **MAINTAIN THE CIRCLES IN YOUR WRISTS, ELBOWS, SHOULDERS, THE SPACE BETWEEN YOUR LEGS, AND KNEES.**

腕肘肩胯膝

104. **WHEN YOU TAKE A STEP YOUR HANDS MOVE CORRESPONDINGLY.**

足踏手腳齊

105. **WHEN ALL YOUR JOINTS ARE JOINED OR CONNECTED THE INNER STRENGTH MOVES THROUGH THEM.**

節節力貫串

106. **WHEN YOU ARE TRAINED, THERE WILL BE NO CRACKS IN YOUR ARMOR.**

處處無乘隙

107. **WHEN INHALING AND EXHALING, YOUR BREATH IS FINE, SOFT, AND CONTINUOUS.**

呼吸細綿綿

108. **WHETHER YOUR MOVEMENT IS SLOW OR FAST, YOUR BREATHING WILL RISE AND FALL NATURALLY.**

升降緩而急

109. WHEN THIS [BREATHING] METHOD IS ACQUIRED, YOU CAN RESPOND TO ANY CHANGE.

得法可應變

110. TO HAVE BOTH THE ART [WISDOM] AND ITS METHODS [TECHNIQUES] IS RARE.

有術方為奇

111. METHOD AND ART ARE TWO AND YET ONE.

法術二而一

112. IF THERE IS BUT A SINGLE WEAKNESS YOU WILL NOT BE ABLE TO WITHSTAND AN OPPONENT.

缺一不能立

113. RAISE BOTH HANDS LIGHTLY.

兩手輕輕起

114. CONTINUOUSLY BEND AND STRETCH WITHOUT INTERRUPTION.

曲伸無斷續

115. ALL YOUR TURNING AND SHIFTING FOLLOWS CURVES.

轉移有曲折

116. THE FORM MOVEMENTS RESEMBLE A ROAMING DRAGON AT PLAY.

形似遊龍戲

117. YOUR MOVEMENT CAN RISE UP VERTICALLY OR BE FLAT ON THE GROUND.

縱橫起與伏

118. THE MOVEMENT BACK AND FORTH BETWEEN YIN AND YANG IS AN ART.

陰陽運行數

119. WHERE THE MIND (INTENT) GOES THE QI IMMEDIATELY FOLLOWS.

意動氣相隨

120. CONNECTING THE JOINTS MAKES THE STORAGE OF STRENGTH TANGIBLE OR REAL.

關節含蓄力

121. STRETCHING YOUR JOINTS ACTIVATES AND ENLIVENS THE BLOOD VESSELS.

舒筋活血脈

122. BY PROTECTING YOUR BLOOD [WITH QI], YOU WILL ATTAIN HEALTH AND SUCCEED IN BEING FIT.

榮衛得適宜

123. WHEN YOU INHALE THE QI RISES [TO THE TOP OF THE HEAD].

一吸氣便提

124. THEN DESCENDS TO RETURN TO THE DANTIEN [ABDOMEN].

氣下可歸臍

125. ONCE THE CHI RISES, SWALLOW ON ITS RETURN TO THE DANTIEN.

一提氣便咽

126. FIRE FROM ABOVE AND WATER FROM BELOW MEET HARMONIOUSLY.

水火得相見

127. A COMPLETE INVESTIGATION IS NECESSARY TO THOROUGHLY UNDERSTAND THE ESSENCE OF THIS ACHIEVEMENT [KUNG FU] THAT IS BOTH INTERNAL AND EXTERNAL.

精研內外功

128. EMPTY YOUR MIND (HEART) AND REINFORCE YOUR ABDOMEN [TO ACHIEVE ENLIGHTENMENT].

心虛腹要實

129. SEIZE YOUR OPPORTUNITY TO CONTROL THE SITUATION.

牽然取其勢

130. THE BEGINNING AND ENDING ARE INSEPARABLE.

首尾不相離

131. OPPOSITES (ORDINARY/EXTRAORDINARY) ARE NECESSARY TO ACHIEVE A MUTUAL FUNCTION.

奇正得相宜

132. IN MOVEMENT AND IN STILLNESS, FOLLOW YOUR HEART'S DESIRE.

動靜隨心欲

133. THIS ENDS THE FIVE CHARACTER SECRETS OF LI DONGFENG.

麤成五字訣

134. TAKE CARE TO STUDY IT CAREFULLY AND DO NOT TAKE IT LIGHTLY.

後學莫輕視

The Five Character Secrets of Li Dongfeng

Anami: without name, nameless. A region beyond the worlds of duality; because this region is without comparatives, there was no way to describe or name it.

Bagua, Baguazhang: A style of Chinese martial art belonging to the Internal School. The name means Eight Trigram Palms.

Beginner's Mind: mind that has no preconceptions or attitudes; a fertile ground for planting new ideas and concepts free from social convention.

Chen Tuan (陳摶): 871-989 A.D. The Daoist Sage who created Liuhebafa, Taiji Ruler, and other qigong methods. His influence was felt among both Confucians and Daoists.

Chen Tunan (陳圖南): A name of Chen Tuan

Chen Yiren (陳亦人): 1909-1982 A.D. One of the Liuhebafa masters who brought the art to Hong Kong in the early 1950's.

Jing Wu Martial Arts Association (精武會): A prestigious organization that fostered the spreading of Taiji among the people of China after the Nationalist Revolution.

Citadel: The Solar Plexus or Heart Center that is emphasized in the methods of Liuhebafa as the energy center from which you issue energy or power.

Crown Chakra: The thousand-petal lotus, the energy center at the top of the head where the Masters long taught as the easiest place to be able to externalize your consciousness.

Dao De Jing: The famous work by Lao Zi that is the basic canon for Daoists

Daoism (Taoism): An ancient teaching on the way of return to the Original Source. This teaching was expressed in the *Dao De Jing* by Lao Zi.

Han Xingyuan (韓星垣): A famous Yiquan master who influenced Li Zhong in his exploration of Liuhebafa.

Heart Center: Also known as the Solar Plexus, this is the center from which energy is issued. This is the point through which you sense and influence the world around you. It is through this center that you place your intent to establish and fulfill your goal or desire.

Hua Shan (華山): One of Daoism's five holy mountains located in north central China. The name means the flowery or beautiful mountain. It is also called the western holy mountain where Chen Tuan spent over thirty years in hermitage.

Immortal (Xian Ren, 仙人): An inevitable state of consciousness for all beings. One who has truly realized who and what they are and now work in harmony with the Life Force.

Jia Desheng: Chen Tuan's student who carved out a cave that would be his master's last earthly home.

King of the Hard Style: Li Zhong's title when he was competing in the external method.

Lao Zi (老子): Author of the Dao De Jing the canon of Daoism.

Li Li (李梨): Lineage student of Song Yuan Tong

Li Zhong (李忠): 1903-1982 A.D. A master of Liuhebafa who popularized the art in the 1970's in the United States.

Li Dongfeng (李東風): A scholar and martial artist at the beginning of the Yuan Dynasty who discovered Chen Tuan's manuscripts on Liuhebafa, mastered the art, and taught it to his followers.

Liu Kun: Lineage student of Song Yuan Tong

Liuhebafaquan (六合八法拳): Chinese martial art belonging to the Internal School. The name means Six Combination Eight Method Boxing.

Main Form: The main practice exercise of Liuhebafa. A series of 66 linked sets consisting of over 360 movements and 700 martial applications. The practice speed of the form can be slow and continuous, alternately fast and slow, or fast.

Majestic Greatness: This is the Void, the Original Source from which all life and energy flows.

Mantis: A Chinese martial art of the External School. Its movements are patterned after a mantis.

Mind/Intent: The creative imagination.

Mount Yun (Yun Shan 雲山): A mountain along the Silk Route in north central China. Li Dongfeng's home and where he taught Liuhebafa after his return from Hua Shan. It means the cloudy or misty mountain.

Mysterious Pass: The neutral point between yin/yang within you where you understand your power of creativity.

Nei Gong (內功): Inner work.

Qing Dynasty: 1644-1911 A.D. The last Chinese dynasty.

Righteousness: The embodiment of the virtues of ethics and morality in service to others.

Shaolin (少林): A Chinese martial art that many call the root of all Chinese martial art. Attributed to the monk Bodhidharma at the Shaolin monastery. Over the centuries, monks spent many years perfecting both external and internal forms of martial art. Many of the Buddhist standing postures influenced the nei gong methods of Liuhebafa.

Sichuan (四川): A province in central China.

Solar Plexus: see Heart Center

Song (鬆): A state of dynamically alive relaxation.

Song Dynasty (宋朝): 960-1279 A.D. Period in which Chen Tuan perfected his dream techniques and influenced Chinese philosophy.

Song Yuan Tong (宋元通): Lineage student of Li Dongfeng.

Stillness: The calm, quiet place within where you meet yourself and listen to celestial music.

Sun Zi (Sun Wu 孫女（孫武）): A Chinese Warrior philosopher that over two thousand years ago compiled a book of strategy, *The Art of War*.

Taijiquan (太極拳): A style of Chinese martial art belonging to the Internal School. The name means grand ultimate.

Taiji Ruler: A qigong exercise set that uses a short dowel to help focus attention and maintain alignments.

Taoism (Daoism): An ancient teaching on the way of return to the Original Source. This teaching was expressed in the *Dao De Jing* by Lao Zi.

Third Eye: The microcosmic energy center that is located behind your eyes between your ears in the center of your head.

True Self: That which you truly are that some call Soul.

Twelve Pillar Standing Postures in Three Levels: Standing postures used to develop inner strength.

Wai Gong (外功): Exercises used to strengthen and fortify the physical body.

Wheel of Awagawan: The cycle of life and rebirth for purification and education.

Wu Yihui (吳翼翬): 1887-1961 A.D. A Liuhebafa master who openly taught the art in Shanghai and Nanjing.

Wudang Mountain (武當山): A famous Daoist enclave in central China.

Xingyiquan (形意拳): A Chinese martial art that belongs to the Internal School. The name means that the movements come out of one's intent.

Xinyi (心意): A Chinese martial art that belongs to the Internal School. The name means mind and imagination combined.

Xiyi (Chen Xiyi 希夷 (陳希夷)): A name given to Chen Tuan by the second Song emperor. It means unfathomable.

Yi Jing (易經): A Chinese classic that uses the combinations of *yin/yang* to express the different forms of experiences and life. The book is usually called the *Book of Changes*.

Yin/Yang (陰陽): The negative and positive energies that combine to produce all things.

Yuan Dynasty (元朝): 1279-1368 A.D. Period when Li Dongfeng discovered Chen Tuan's manuscripts of Liuhebafa.

Zhang Jishan (張繼善): Lineage student of Song Yuan Tong.

Zhang Xueli (張學禮): Lineage student of Song Yuan Tong.

Zhao Guangyi (趙光義 (太宗)): r. 976-997, the second Song emperor called Taizong.

Zhao Kuanyin (趙匡胤 (太祖)): r. 960-976, the first Song emperor called Taizu.

Index

101 REFLECTIONS ON TAI CHI CHUAN
108 INSIGHTS INTO TAI CHI CHUAN
A SUDDEN DAWN: THE EPIC JOURNEY OF BODHIDHARMA
A WOMAN'S QIGONG GUIDE
ADVANCING IN TAE KWON DO
ANALYSIS OF SHAOLIN CHIN NA 2ND ED
ANCIENT CHINESE WEAPONS
THE ART AND SCIENCE OF STAFF FIGHTING
THE ART AND SCIENCE OF STICK FIGHTING
ART OF HOJO UNDO
ARTHRITIS RELIEF, 3D ED.
BACK PAIN RELIEF, 2ND ED.
BAGUAZHANG, 2ND ED.
BRAIN FITNESS
CARDIO KICKBOXING ELITE
CHIN NA IN GROUND FIGHTING
CHINESE FAST WRESTLING
CHINESE FITNESS
CHINESE TUI NA MASSAGE
CHOJUN
COMPLETE MARTIAL ARTIST
COMPREHENSIVE APPLICATIONS OF SHAOLIN CHIN NA
CONFLICT COMMUNICATION
CROCODILE AND THE CRANE: A NOVEL
CUTTING SEASON: A XENON PEARL MARTIAL ARTS THRILLER
DAO DE JING
DAO IN ACTION
DEFENSIVE TACTICS
DESHI: A CONNOR BURKE MARTIAL ARTS THRILLER
DIRTY GROUND
DR. WU'S HEAD MASSAGE
DUKKHA HUNGRY GHOSTS
DUKKHA REVERB
DUKKHA, THE SUFFERING: AN EYE FOR AN EYE
DUKKHA UNLOADED
ENZAN: THE FAR MOUNTAIN, A CONNOR BURKE MARTIAL ARTS
    THRILLER
ESSENCE OF SHAOLIN WHITE CRANE
EVEN IF IT KILLS ME
EXPLORING TAI CHI
FACING VIOLENCE
FIGHT BACK
FIGHT LIKE A PHYSICIST
THE FIGHTER'S BODY
FIGHTER'S FACT BOOK
FIGHTER'S FACT BOOK 2
THE FIGHTING ARTS
FIGHTING THE PAIN RESISTANT ATTACKER
FIRST DEFENSE
FORCE DECISIONS: A CITIZENS GUIDE
FOX BORROWS THE TIGER'S AWE
INSIDE TAI CHI
THE JUDO ADVANTAGE
THE JUJI GATAME ENCYCLOPEDIA
KAGE: THE SHADOW, A CONNOR BURKE MARTIAL ARTS THRILLER
KARATE SCIENCE
KATA AND THE TRANSMISSION OF KNOWLEDGE
KRAV MAGA COMBATIVES
KRAV MAGA PROFESSIONAL TACTICS
KRAV MAGA WEAPON DEFENSES
LITTLE BLACK BOOK OF VIOLENCE
LIUHEBAFA FIVE CHARACTER SECRETS
MARTIAL ARTS ATHLETE
MARTIAL ARTS INSTRUCTION
MARTIAL WAY AND ITS VIRTUES
MASK OF THE KING
MEDITATIONS ON VIOLENCE
MERIDIAN QIGONG EXERCISES
MIND/BODY FITNESS
MINDFUL EXERCISE
THE MIND INSIDE TAI CHI
THE MIND INSIDE YANG STYLE TAI CHI CHUAN
MUGAI RYU
NATURAL HEALING WITH QIGONG
NORTHERN SHAOLIN SWORD, 2ND ED.
OKINAWA'S COMPLETE KARATE SYSTEM: ISSHIN RYU
THE PAIN-FREE BACK

PAIN-FREE JOINTS
POWER BODY
PRINCIPLES OF TRADITIONAL CHINESE MEDICINE
THE PROTECTOR ETHIC
QIGONG FOR HEALTH & MARTIAL ARTS 2ND ED.
QIGONG FOR LIVING
QIGONG FOR TREATING COMMON AILMENTS
QIGONG MASSAGE
QIGONG MEDITATION: EMBRYONIC BREATHING
QIGONG MEDITATION: SMALL CIRCULATION
QIGONG, THE SECRET OF YOUTH: DA MO'S CLASSICS
QUIET TEACHER: A XENON PEARL MARTIAL ARTS THRILLER
RAVEN'S WARRIOR
REDEMPTION
ROOT OF CHINESE QIGONG, 2ND ED.
SAMBO ENCYCLOPEDIA
SCALING FORCE
SELF-DEFENSE FOR WOMEN
SENSEI: A CONNOR BURKE MARTIAL ARTS THRILLER
SHIHAN TE: THE BUNKAI OF KATA
SHIN GI TAI: KARATE TRAINING FOR BODY, MIND, AND SPIRIT
SIMPLE CHINESE MEDICINE
SIMPLE QIGONG EXERCISES FOR HEALTH, 3RD ED.
SIMPLIFIED TAI CHI CHUAN, 2ND ED.
SOLO TRAINING
SOLO TRAINING 2
SPOTTING DANGER BEFORE DANGER SPOTS YOU
SUMO FOR MIXED MARTIAL ARTS
SUNRISE TAI CHI
SUNSET TAI CHI
SURVIVING ARMED ASSAULTS
TAE KWON DO: THE KOREAN MARTIAL ART
TAEKWONDO BLACK BELT POOMSAE
TAEKWONDO: A PATH TO EXCELLENCE
TAEKWONDO: ANCIENT WISDOM FOR THE MODERN WARRIOR
TAEKWONDO: DEFENSE AGAINST WEAPONS
TAEKWONDO: SPIRIT AND PRACTICE
TAO OF BIOENERGETICS
TAI CHI BALL QIGONG: FOR HEALTH AND MARTIAL ARTS
TAI CHI BALL WORKOUT FOR BEGINNERS
THE TAI CHI BOOK
TAI CHI CHIN NA: THE SEIZING ART OF TAI CHI CHUAN,
    2ND ED.
TAI CHI CHUAN CLASSICAL YANG STYLE, 2ND ED.
TAI CHI CHUAN MARTIAL POWER, 3RD ED.
TAI CHI CONNECTIONS
TAI CHI DYNAMICS
TAI CHI FOR DEPRESSION
TAI CHI IN 10 WEEKS
TAI CHI QIGONG, 3RD ED.
TAI CHI SECRETS OF THE ANCIENT MASTERS
TAI CHI SECRETS OF THE WU & LI STYLES
TAI CHI SECRETS OF THE WU STYLE
TAI CHI SECRETS OF THE YANG STYLE
TAI CHI SWORD: CLASSICAL YANG STYLE, 2ND ED.
TAI CHI SWORD FOR BEGINNERS
TAI CHI WALKING
TAIJIQUAN THEORY OF DR. YANG, JWING-MING
TAO OF BIOENERGETICS
TENGU: THE MOUNTAIN GOBLIN, A CONNOR BURKE MARTIAL ARTS
    THRILLER
TIMING IN THE FIGHTING ARTS
TRADITIONAL CHINESE HEALTH SECRETS
TRADITIONAL TAEKWONDO
TRAINING FOR SUDDEN VIOLENCE
TRUE WELLNESS
TRUE WELLNESS: THE MIND
TRUE WELLNESS FOR YOUR HEART
THE WARRIOR'S MANIFESTO
WAY OF KATA
WAY OF KENDO AND KENJITSU
WAY OF SANCHIN KATA
WAY TO BLACK BELT
WESTERN HERBS FOR MARTIAL ARTISTS
WILD GOOSE QIGONG
WINNING FIGHTS
WISDOM'S WAY
XINGYIQUAN

DVDS FROM YMAA

ADVANCED PRACTICAL CHIN NA IN-DEPTH
ANALYSIS OF SHAOLIN CHIN NA
ATTACK THE ATTACK
BAGUA FOR BEGINNERS 1
BAGUA FOR BEGINNERS 2
BAGUAZHANG: EMEI BAGUAZHANG
BEGINNER QIGONG FOR WOMEN 1
BEGINNER QIGONG FOR WOMEN 2
BEGINNER TAI CHI FOR HEALTH
CHEN STYLE TAIJIQUAN
CHEN TAI CHI FOR BEGINNERS
CHIN NA IN-DEPTH COURSES 1—4
CHIN NA IN-DEPTH COURSES 5—8
CHIN NA IN-DEPTH COURSES 9—12
FACING VIOLENCE: 7 THINGS A MARTIAL ARTIST MUST KNOW
FIVE ANIMAL SPORTS
FIVE ELEMENTS ENERGY BALANCE
INFIGHTING
INTRODUCTION TO QI GONG FOR BEGINNERS
JOINT LOCKS
KNIFE DEFENSE: TRADITIONAL TECHNIQUES AGAINST A DAGGER
KUNG FU BODY CONDITIONING 1
KUNG FU BODY CONDITIONING 2
KUNG FU FOR KIDS
KUNG FU FOR TEENS
LOGIC OF VIOLENCE
MERIDIAN QIGONG
NEIGONG FOR MARTIAL ARTS
NORTHERN SHAOLIN SWORD : SAN CAI JIAN, KUN WU JIAN, QI MEN JIAN
QI GONG 30-DAY CHALLENGE
QI GONG FOR ANXIETY
QI GONG FOR ARMS, WRISTS, AND HANDS
QIGONG FOR BEGINNERS: FRAGRANCE
QI GONG FOR BETTER BREATHING
QI GONG FOR CANCER
QI GONG FOR ENERGY AND VITALITY
QI GONG FOR HEADACHES
QI GONG FOR HEALING
QI GONG FOR HEALTHY JOINTS
QI GONG FOR HIGH BLOOD PRESSURE
QIGONG FOR LONGEVITY
QI GONG FOR STRONG BONES
QI GONG FOR THE UPPER BACK AND NECK
QIGONG FOR WOMEN
QIGONG FOR WOMEN WITH DAISY LEE
QIGONG MASSAGE
QIGONG MINDFULNESS IN MOTION
QIGONG: 15 MINUTES TO HEALTH
SABER FUNDAMENTAL TRAINING
SAI TRAINING AND SEQUENCES
SANCHIN KATA: TRADITIONAL TRAINING FOR KARATE POWER
SCALING FORCE
SHAOLIN KUNG FU FUNDAMENTAL TRAINING: COURSES 1 & 2
SHAOLIN LONG FIST KUNG FU: ADVANCED SEQUENCES 1
SHAOLIN LONG FIST KUNG FU: ADVANCED SEQUENCES 2
SHAOLIN LONG FIST KUNG FU: BASIC SEQUENCES
SHAOLIN LONG FIST KUNG FU: INTERMEDIATE SEQUENCES
SHAOLIN SABER: BASIC SEQUENCES
SHAOLIN STAFF: BASIC SEQUENCES
SHAOLIN WHITE CRANE GONG FU BASIC TRAINING: COURSES 1 & 2
SHAOLIN WHITE CRANE GONG FU BASIC TRAINING: COURSES 3 & 4

SHUAI JIAO: KUNG FU WRESTLING
SIMPLE QIGONG EXERCISES FOR HEALTH
SIMPLE QIGONG EXERCISES FOR ARTHRITIS RELIEF
SIMPLE QIGONG EXERCISES FOR BACK PAIN RELIEF
SIMPLIFIED TAI CHI CHUAN: 24 & 48 POSTURES
SIMPLIFIED TAI CHI FOR BEGINNERS 48
SUNRISE TAI CHI
SUNSET TAI CHI
SWORD: FUNDAMENTAL TRAINING
TAEKWONDO KORYO POOMSAE
TAI CHI BALL QIGONG: COURSES 1 & 2
TAI CHI BALL QIGONG: COURSES 3 & 4
TAI CHI BALL WORKOUT FOR BEGINNERS
TAI CHI CHUAN CLASSICAL YANG STYLE
TAI CHI CONNECTIONS
TAI CHI ENERGY PATTERNS
TAI CHI FIGHTING SET
TAI CHI FIT: 24 FORM
TAI CHI FIT: FLOW
TAI CHI FIT: FUSION BAMBOO
TAI CHI FIT: FUSION FIRE
TAI CHI FIT: FUSION IRON
TAI CHI FIT: HEART HEALTH WORKOUT
TAI CHI FIT IN PARADISE
TAI CHI FIT: OVER 50
TAI CHI FIT OVER 50: BALANCE EXERCISES
TAI CHI FIT OVER 50: SEATED WORKOUT
TAI CHI FIT OVER 60: GENTLE EXERCISES
TAI CHI FIT OVER 60: HEALTHY JOINTS
TAI CHI FIT OVER 60: LIVE LONGER
TAI CHI FIT: STRENGTH
TAI CHI FIT: TO GO
TAI CHI FOR WOMEN
TAI CHI FUSION: FIRE
TAI CHI QIGONG
TAI CHI PUSHING HANDS: COURSES 1 & 2
TAI CHI PUSHING HANDS: COURSES 3 & 4
TAI CHI SWORD: CLASSICAL YANG STYLE
TAI CHI SWORD FOR BEGINNERS
TAI CHI SYMBOL: YIN YANG STICKING HANDS
TAIJI & SHAOLIN STAFF: FUNDAMENTAL TRAINING
TAIJI CHIN NA IN-DEPTH
TAIJI 37 POSTURES MARTIAL APPLICATIONS
TAIJI SABER CLASSICAL YANG STYLE
TAIJI WRESTLING
TRAINING FOR SUDDEN VIOLENCE
UNDERSTANDING QIGONG 1: WHAT IS QI? • HUMAN QI
    CIRCULATORY SYSTEM
UNDERSTANDING QIGONG 2: KEY POINTS • QIGONG BREATHING
UNDERSTANDING QIGONG 3: EMBRYONIC BREATHING
UNDERSTANDING QIGONG 4: FOUR SEASONS QIGONG
UNDERSTANDING QIGONG 5: SMALL CIRCULATION
UNDERSTANDING QIGONG 6: MARTIAL QIGONG BREATHING
WATER STYLE FOR BEGINNERS
WHITE CRANE HARD & SOFT QIGONG
YANG TAI CHI FOR BEGINNERSS
WUDANG KUNG FU: FUNDAMENTAL TRAINING
WUDANG SWORD
WUDANG TAIJIQUAN
XINGYIQUAN
YANG TAI CHI FOR BEGINNERS

more products available from . . .

YMAA Publication Center, Inc. 楊氏東方文化出版中心

1-800-669-8892 • info@ymaa.com • www.ymaa.com